Skills and Protocols in Obstetrics and Gynaecology

For Students, Trainees and Practitioners

Rubina Sohail

©

Paramount Books (Pvt.) Ltd.

Karachi | Lahore | Islamabad | Sukkur | Faisalabad | Peshawar | Abbottabad

Skills and Protocols in Obstetrics and Gynaecology

by

Rubina Sohail

Medical knowledge is constantly changing. As new information becomes available, changes in treatment, procedures, equipment and the use of drugs become necessary. The editors, contributors and the publishers have, as far as it is possible, taken care to ensure that the information given in this text is accurate and up-to-date. However, readers are strongly advised to confirm that the information, especially with regard to drug usage, complies with the latest legislation and standards of practice. Neither the publisher nor the authors assume any responsibility for any loss or injury and/or damage to person or property arising out of or related to any use of the material contained in this handbook.

First Edition 2016

Paramount Books (Pvt.) Ltd.

152/O, Block-2, P.E.C.H.S., Karachi-75400. Tel: 34310030
Fax: 34553772, E-mail: info@paramountbooks.com.pk
Website: www.paramountbooks.com.pk

ISBN: 978-969-637-116-8

Printed in Pakistan

Foreword

It gives me great pleasure in writing the foreword of this book written by Professor Rubina Sohail. TOACS was introduced to replace viva because table viva previously used for assessment in the postgraduate examination carried a lot of subjectivity on the part of examiners and there was no standardization regarding questions and answers. The new system of TOACS is meant to take away subjectivity from the final assessment of postgraduate candidates and introduce a modern system of predetermined questions, answers, and instructions regarding the awarding of marks. Unfortunately, there is very little emphasis on this component, in the preparation of postgraduate students, which would prepare them for such kind of assessment.

Professor Rubina, has been an examiner of FCPS and other postgraduate diplomas for a long time and is one of the most experienced teachers and assessors at the highest level of examination in our country. She has conducted TOACS courses for many years and has mastered the way a candidate should prepare for this part of evaluation in their final assessment. The courses run by Professor Rubina are popular from Karachi to Peshawar, to such an extent that every time she announces a course, a large number of candidates, many a times, more than a hundred register for the course fully realizing the importance of this exercise. In writing the present book, Rubina has made appreciable use of her knowledge and experience in presenting the required information, clearly and concisely.

I have scanned the book and found it extremely useful particularly from the point of view of the students. She has judiciously picked up important topics regarding skills, protocols, and standard operating procedures and has put forth this information deftly, making the task easy to follow and the job of the learner simpler. This book is a suitable resource for students and doctors to master their skills and some aspects of patient management. I found the section about protocols particularly interesting, because this information has not been presented in any other book, in this fashion. I am sure the students, trainees and young doctors will find the information practical and handy for good clinical practice.

I very strongly recommend this book to all medical students, postgraduate trainees and young doctors and hope that the book will become a popular handbook for all the Obstetrics and Gynaecology residents working in various institutions of the country.

I have been always been requesting my colleagues to write textbooks or handbooks like this to help our students but generally, only a very few people have made an effort in writing books for postgraduate students. I must compliment Rubina, for making this effort, which I know will go a long way in helping our students.

In the end I must compliment Rubina once again, for her endeavour in writing this useful book for our postgraduate students, which is the need of the time and I hope that she continues to contribute more books like this and also comes out with a textbook because in Pakistan there is a dearth of books coming out from teaching institutions.

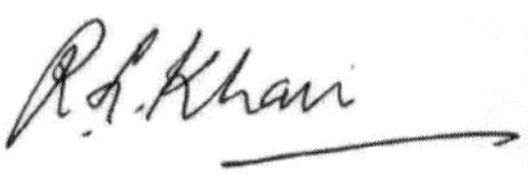

Prof. Rashid Latif Khan

Professor Emeritus

Contents

Dedicated to

my mother, Dr Razia Sajjad
who believed in promoting education,
specially for women

Preface

This book is an endeavour to put my passion for teaching to good use for students who are not clear as to how to go about learning skills. Most of the students start learning skills at the end of their training, as part of preparations for their examination. I recommend reading and applying material from this book, starting from the early part of the training so that enough opportunity exists to practice the skills learnt again and again.

This book contains sections on skills, standard operating procedures, protocols and guidelines adapted from RCOG for local use. The book is directed towards MBBS students, postgraduate trainees of MCPS, FCPS, DGO, MS, and MRCOG and young doctors. Learning a skill is not possible unless the theory of performing the skill is not mastered prior to the actual procedure. Therefore, twenty three skills have been given in the form of a checklist. The checklist helps in concisely putting forward each task in the correct sequence. Adapted RCOG guidelines are easy to read and remember to be applied in clinical situations. The standard operating procedures clarify exactly what and how things need to be done.

I am sure both students and doctors will find the book useful not only for passing the examination, but also for helping them, To become better doctors. I look forward to feedback and advice on how to make this book more useful and effective.

Acknowledgement

I would like to express my gratitude to the many people who saw me through this book; the list is long and I sincerely hope, I do not miss out anybody. I thank all, who provided support and assisted in editing and proofreading of this book. I would specially like to mention and thank my colleagues and trainees in unit II and III of the Department of Obstetrics and Gynaecology at the Services Institute of Medical Sciences, Lahore. Their hard work, support, critical evaluation and feedback were indispensable to this exercise. I would particularly like to mention doctors Saima Iqbal, Asifa Naureen, Khadija Asim, Asma Mushtaq, Shazia Ashfaque, Rukhsana, Sofia Tabbasum, and Aqeela Abbas among others for their efforts.

I am indebted to Professor Rashid Latif Khan for his encouragement and support, Professor Farrukh Zaman for believing in my abilities, Professor Sohail Khurshid Lodhi for the crisp feedback and my sons Daniyal and Raza for their appreciation and reminding me of the nuances of academic writing. I would specially like to thank the chairman of the guidelines committee of Royal College of Obstetricians and Gynaecologists and his team for their facilitation and allowing adaptation of RCOG guidelines for local use.

The list of acknowledgements will not be complete without thanking and appreciating the efforts of Mr Ghazzanfar Ali, my assistant for patiently bearing with me and endlessly modifying text and correcting errors. I thank my publishers Paramount Books (Pvt.) Ltd. for their contribution in making this a reality.

Lastly, I would like to acknowledge my students and junior colleagues, who brighten up my day and make this effort worthwhile.

Rubina Sohail

List of Abbreviations

Abbreviation	Definition
IUCD	Intra Uterine Contraceptive Device
USG	Ultrasonography
CTG	Cardiotocography
IV	Intravenous
L/S	Lecithin Sphingomyelin Ratio
FHR	Foetal Heart Rate
ECV	External Cephalic Version
IUD	Intra Uterine Demise
PV	Per Vaginal
AP	Antero Posterior
EFW	Estimated Foetal Weight
OA	Occipito Anterior
PPICD	Postpartum Intra Uterine Contraceptive Device
NSAID	Non-steroidal Anti-inflammatory Drug
ACOG	American College of Obstetricians and Gynaecologists
BP	Blood Pressure
C/S	Caesarean Section
ICU	Intensive Care Unit
ECG	Electrocardiogram
IM	Intra Muscular
BPP	Biophysical Profile
SR	Senior Registrar
SOS	SI Opus Sit (if it is necessary)
CBC	Complete Blood Count
BSR	Blood Sugar Random
C/E	Complete Examination
SVD	Spontaneous Vaginal Delivery
AFI	Amniotic Fluid Index
MOD	Mode of Delivery

QID	Quarter in Die (four times a day)
TLC	Total Leukocyte Count
CPD	Cephalo Pelvic Disproportion
ALT	Alanine Transaminases
AST	Aspartate Transaminases
MgSo4	Magnesium Sulphate
LFT	Liver Function Tests
RFT	Renal Function Tests
N/S	Normal Saline
HIV	Human Immuno-deficiency Virus
HAART	Highly Active Antiretroviral Therapy
PPH	Postpartum Haemorrhage
NICU	Neonatal Intensive Care Unit
IUGR	Intra Uterine Growth Restriction
OBG	Obstetrics
FPU	Foetoplacental Unit
VBAC	Vaginal Birth After Caesarean Section
DVT	Deep Vein Thrombosis
TOLAC	Trail of Labour After Previous Caesarean Delivery
ZDB	Zidovudine
PCP	Pneumocystis Pneumonia
DNA	Deoxyribonucleic Acid
CPR	Cardio Pulmonary Resuscitation
PPROM	Preterm Prelabour Rupture of Membrane
EOGBS	Early Onset Neonatal Group B Streptococcal
GBS	Group B Streptococcal

SECTION 01

SKILLS

Introduction to Skills

Mother of All Skills—How to Develop a Skill?

This has been written to guide the learner/trainee in "How to develop a skill". In the process, if the correct order is followed, the skill will be mastered in easy steps. The following order should be followed:

1. Be clear about the **objective**.
2. **Allocate time** in your schedule to learn.
3. **Background knowledge** related to achieve the desired skill is essential. As an example: In order to perform an appendicectomy one must know the anatomy of the anterior abdominal wall and the variations in the type of the appendix.
4. A **theory of the steps** to achieve the skill is essential. In this book an effort has been made so that the theoretical steps needed to learn the skills are available. These can be learnt by heart and mastered
5. Identify the **correct technique** to begin with. Do not worry about not being able to do it in the first attempt.
6. **Break the task** into smaller components.
7. **Speak and perform:** It is recommended that when the skill is being performed, one should speak out the theoretical steps, aloud, at the same time.
8. **Repetition** with the correct technique is the key. Keep on repeating the theory and the practice of the task with the correct technique again and again.
9. It is preferable to **learn on a dummy** and then move on to live subjects, learn initially under supervision and then independently.
10. One may not realize what mistake(s) one is making and repetition with any wrong step may be a hindrance in achieving accuracy. As an incorrect bowling style may result in delivering no balls. **Avoid making mistakes.**
11. **Focus on accuracy.** Each time you perform the task, try not to make any mistake. Remember playing marbles or netball in school. As an

example: The objective is to hit the desired marble only, without hitting any other marble lying in close vicinity in order to win the game. This could happen by chance, but the champion (pockets full of marbles) would be was the boy who could do it *almost* every time.

12. **Apply** your newly acquired skills to your work.
13. If you do not do this, the skills may wame and you may lose confidence. Moreover this is the reason why you acquired the given skills.
14. **Demonstrate** your skills to colleagues.
15. **Teach others** (colleagues, friend's, students, etc.). This is probably the best way to learn.

Components of Examination Trolley 01

GENERAL RESOURCES	
Examination table.	
Light source.	
Height scale.	
Weight scale.	
GENERAL PHYSICAL EXAMINATION	
Stethoscope.	
B.P. apparatus.	
Torch.	
Tongue depressor.	
Hammer.	
Watch with seconds needle.	
OBSTETRICAL EXAMINATION	
Two draw sheets.	
Measuring tape.	
Foetoscope.	
GYNAECOLOGICAL EXAMINATION COMPONENTS OF TROLLEY	
Chittel's forceps with jar.	
Cotton swabs in saline solution.	
Water based gel.	
Kidney tray.	
Cusco speculum.	
Disposable gloves.	
Sanitary pads.	

PAP SMEAR	
Ayres spatula.	
Glass slides.	
Fixative—spray or solution.	
Markers.	
UTEROVAGINAL PROLAPSE EXAMINATION	
Single blade Sims speculum.	
Sponge holding forceps.	
Tenaculum forceps.	

General Physical Examination 02

There are four major components of general physical examination. These comprise the following:	
1. GENERAL APPEARANCE AND ORIENTATION IN TIME AND SPACE	
2. HEIGHT AND WEIGHT (CALCULATE BMI)	
3. VITAL SIGNS	
Pulse.	
Blood pressure.	
Temperature.	
Respiratory rate.	
4. SPECIFIC SIGNS	
Oro-dental hygiene.	
Pallor.	
Thyroid.	
Jaundice.	
Koilonychia.	
Clubbing.	
Cyanosis.	
Lymph nodes.	
Sacral oedema and spine.	
Pedal oedema.	
JVP (In case of cardiac patient only)	
Patellar and ankle reflex (In case of hypertension)	

The above mentioned information is required for general physical examination. However the suggested order of examination to get this information is given in the following paragraph. An important point to be noted over here is that systemic examination has to be performed as well.

For this, a detailed systemic examination is not needed in most of the cases. It is recommended that essential components of systemic examination should be merged with the components of general physical examination and breast examination and the combination of all these three examination should be performed in the following order.

EXAMINE THE FOLLOWING AREAS IN THE PRESCRIBED ORDER:

Hands and arms.	
Head and neck.	
Back and legs.	
1. **Hands and arms.** a. Vital signs. – Temperature. – Pulse. – Blood pressure. – Respiratory rate. b. Koilonychia. c. Clubbing. d. Cyanosis.	
2. **Head and neck.** a. Pallor. b. Jaundice. c. Orodental hygiene. d. Thyroid. e. Lymph nodes. f. JVP.	
3. **Legs and back.** a. Sacral oedema and spine. b. Pedal oedema.	

PALLOR	
Examine both palms, nailbed, conjunctiva of both eyes and under surface of tongue.	
CYANOSIS	
Look for cyanosis on nails tips, tip of nose and lips.	
JAUNDICE	
Jaundice is noted on skin and sclera of both eyes at day time.	
LYMPH NODES	
For palpation of cervical lymph nodes, start palpating submandibular, anterior cervical chain, posterior cervical, supra clavicular, preauricular, and post auricular, sub occipital, lymph nodes.	

03 Breast and Axillary Lymph Nodes Examination

PREREQUISITES	
Introduce and greet the patient.	
Explain the procedure and take verbal consent.	
Reassure and instruct the patient to inform you, if she feels pain.	
Patient's privacy, appropriate light, couch and draw sheets (size: 1'x4' and 2'x4').	
POSITION	
Patient must be sitting on examination couch with arms at side.	
Stand on the patient's right side.	
Proper exposure is necessary. Ideally shirt should be removed.	
PROCEDURE	
INSPECTION	
First inspection. Examine breasts for size, symmetry, shape, contour, skin and scars.	
Second inspection. Ask patient to raise both arms above the head and inspect breasts.	
Third inspection. Ask patient to place both hands on waist and press elbows forward to examine.	
Fourth inspection. Ask patient to lean forward with arms extended in front and examine.	
PALPATION	
Use proper draping technique with patient in sitting position.	

First palpation. Bimanual palpation: Place one hand above, and one hand below the patient's right breast. Gently compress the breast tissue between the pads of your fingertips. Note consistency, nodules, masses, or tenderness.	
Lymph node examination. Patient seated with gown in place. Use index and middle fingers. Press firmly and move the skin over the underlying tissue in a rotatory motion. Note any tenderness or enlargement.	
Palpate the cervical lymph nodes bilaterally.	
Palpate axillary nodes: Place patient's ipsilateral arm on your shoulder. With fingers of opposite hand, reach as high as possible towards the apex of the axilla. Bring your hand down the axilla palpating anteriorly along the edge of the pectorals, and posteriorly along the latissimus (forming a triangle, with the apex at the top). One or two soft, small (<1 cm) nodes may be felt, especially in thin patients. Repeat for the other axilla.	
Step around behind the patient and palpate for supraclavicular nodes.	
Second palpation: Ask the patient to lie down,using palmar surface of first three fingers (rotatory motion) compress the breast tissue gently against the chest wall. Examine the breast in a radial pattern. Note tissue consistency, elasticity, induration, masses or tenderness.	
Palpate axillary tail.	
Palpate the nipples and areola and note the elasticity, discharge, retraction, inversion and flattening of the nipple.	
Gently express nipple using thumb and forefinger and look for discharge.	
POST-PROCEDURE	
Cover and thank the patient.	
DOCUMENTATION	
Document the date, time and relevant information.	

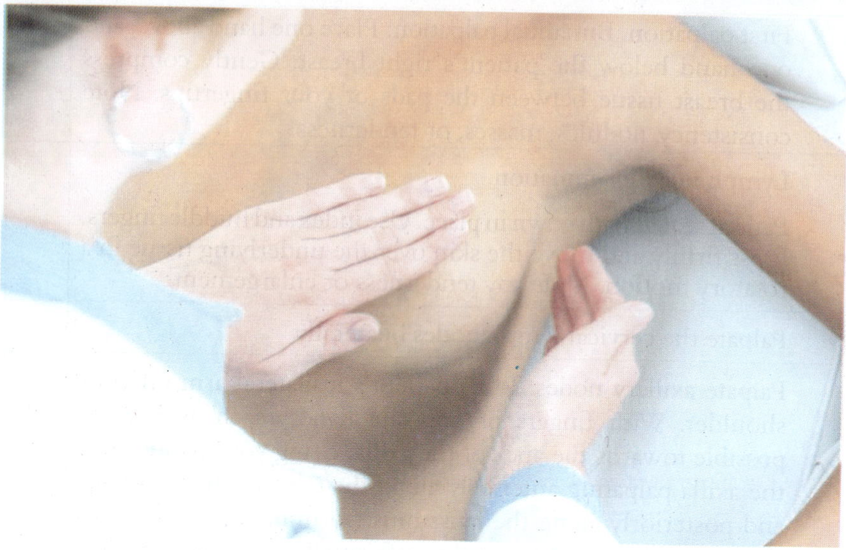

Fig. 3.1 Breast examination

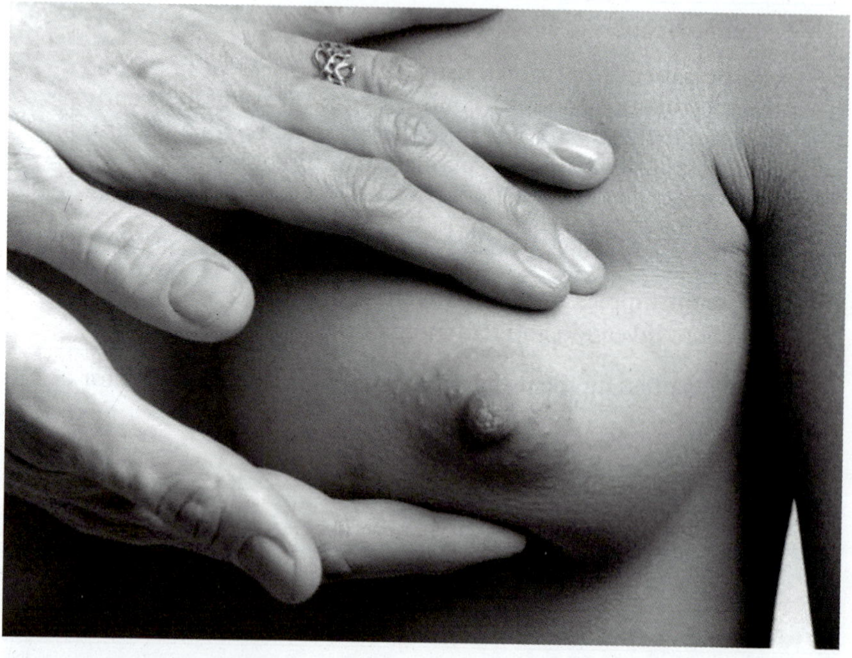

Fig. 3.2 Palpation of breast

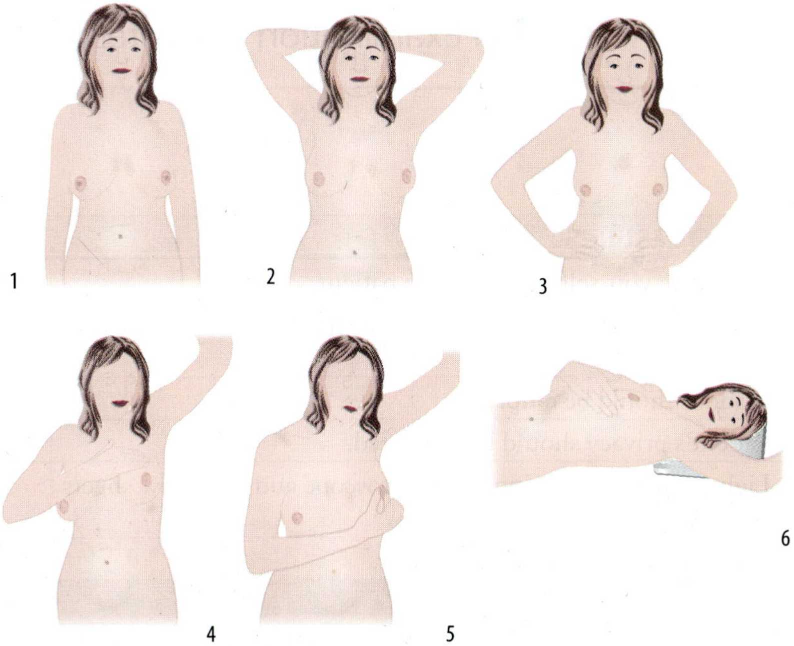

Fig. 3.3 Positions for breast examination

04 Abdominal Examination in Obstetrics

PREREQUISITES	
Introduce yourself and greet the patient.	
Take verbal consent, reassure and instruct her to inform you, if she feels pain.	
Bladder should be empty.	
Patient's privacy should be respected.	
Light, couch, measuring tape, foetoscope and two draw sheets size 1'x4' and 2'x4'.	
Wash hands or clean with sanitizer.	
POSITION OF THE PATIENT	
Semi recumbent position with a wedge under the right buttock.	
DRAPING THE PATIENT	
Stand on the right side of the patient.	
Cover the patient with two draw sheets, one from neck to xiphisternum and the second from knee to pubic symphysis, thus exposing the abdomen.	
PROCEDURE	
INSPECTION	
Note shape of the uterus and any asymmetry.	
Look for enlargement, distension, pigmentation, striaegravidarum or stretch marks—Linea niagra, previous operative (caesarean) scars or any other abnormality and foetal movements.	
PALPATION	
Symphysio-fundal height (cm) measurement: Palpate down from xiphisternum to determine the highest part of the uterine fundus. Mark this point and place a tape measure turned upside down from the mid-point on the uppermost border of the symphysis pubis over the curve of the uterus to the marked point. Turn the tape and record the actual measurement in cm.	

PALPATE USING FOUR LEOPOLD'S MANOEUVRES	
Fundal grip: Both hands are placed over the fundus. A hard smooth, round pole indicates a foetal head. A softer triangular pole continuous with the foetal body is the foetal buttocks (breech).	
Lateral grip: Lie, amount of liquor and weight of baby are assessed by lateral palpation. This manoeuvre determines the site on which the foetal back lies. The palms of the hands are placed on either side of the abdomen. On one side the smooth contour of the back is felt while the other side contains compressible area and nodular parts (limbs).	
Pawliks grip: A single examination hand is placed just above the symphysis to grasp the foetal part that overrides the symphysis between thumb and three fingers. The head is felt as a hard object and in breech presentation, the irregular nodular bottom is felt.	
Pelvic grip: Each hand is placed on either side of the foetal head to determine: The **attitude** of the foetal head. **Engagement of the foetal head**—if the whole head is palpable, it is likely to be free (5/5). When the head is no longer moveable, it has engaged and only 1/5 or 2/5 palpable.	
AUSCULTATION	
Auscultation of fov for one minute by foetoscope.	
POST-PROCEDURE	
Cover and thank the patient.	
Wash hands.	
Document the examination.	
DOCUMENTATION	
Note the date, time and findings of examination.	

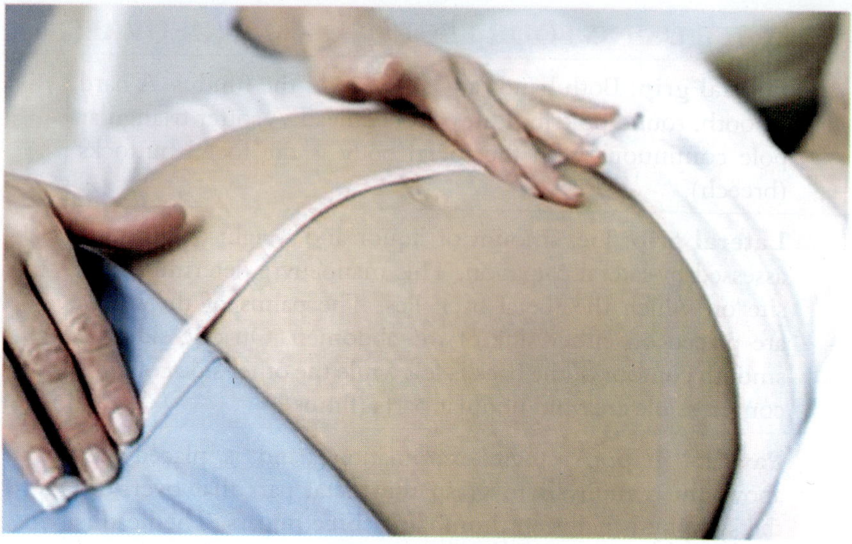

Fig. 4.1 Measurement of symphysio funded height

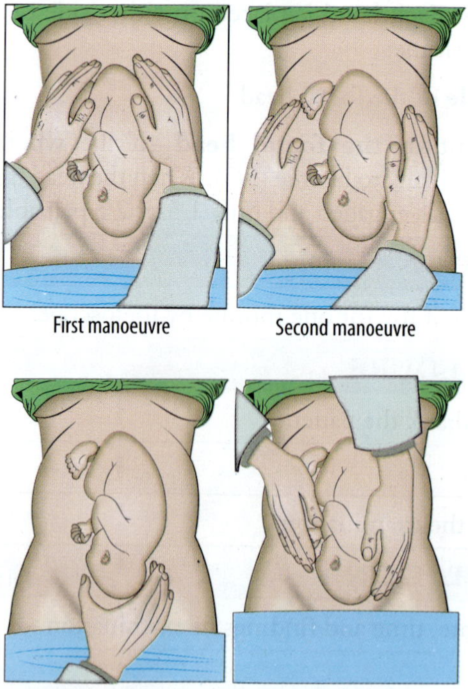

Fig. 4.2 Manoeuvres of abdominal examination

Vaginal Examination 05

PREREQUISITES	
Make introduction and take consent from the patient.	
Explain the procedure and the need for vaginal examination.	
Allay the anxiety of the patient.	
Check examination trolley.	
Instruct the patient to empty the urinary bladder.	
POSITION	
Ask patient to undress and lie in the supine position with legs abducted and flexed at the knees.	
DRAPING	
A draw sheet should be placed covering the thighs upto the knees.Adjust the light.	
Wash hands or clean with sterillium and wear gloves.	
PROCEDURE	
INSPECTION	
Separate the labia majora gently with the index finger and thumb of one gloved hand.	
Inspect and comment on the mons pubis, clitoris, labia majora, labia minora, vestibule, urethral orifice, perineum, peri-anal and anal area.	
Instruct the patient to strain and cough.	
Identify and examine the opening of the Bartholin's gland.	
SPECULUM EXAMINATION	
Select a suitable sized Cusco's speculum.	
Hold the closed blades of the bivalve speculum between the index and middle fingers of the right hand and place the thumb on the upper posterior rim of the speculum.	
Separate the labia majora with the index finger and thumb of the left-gloved hand to expose the vaginal introitus.	

Place the tip of the lubricated speculum at the vaginal introitus, with the blades lying transversely and gently advance the blades of the speculum into the vagina and sliding against the posterior vaginal wall.	
Open the blades of the speculum and fix it. Inspect the vaginal walls.	
Take a pap smear, if needed.	
Gently withdraw the slightly open speculum and once the cervix has been passed, close the blades and withdraw the speculum from the vagina.	
BIMANUAL PALPATION	
Separate the labia majora with the index finger and thumb of the left gloved hand to expose the introitus.	
Insert the index finger of the right gloved hand into the vagina first; then insert the middle finger, when the patient relaxes the muscles around the vagina.	
Palpate the vaginal walls and cervix.	
Place the vaginal fingers in front of the cervix in the anterior fornix and palpate the fornix.	
Place the left hand (abdominal hand) just below the umbilicus and gradually move it lower until the fundus is caught and press against the fingers in the anterior fornix and palpate the uterus. Palpate the right and left adnexae in a similar fashion.	
Place the fingers of the vaginal hand in the posterior fornix and palpate the pouch of Douglas.	
Inspect glove for blood or abnormal discharge.	
RECTOVAGINAL EXAM (WHENEVER INDICATED)	
Insert the index or middle fingers of the right gloved hand into the anal canal and the left hand on the lower abdomen and proceed as in the bimanual vaginal examination.	
Insert the index finger of the right hand in the vagina and the middle finger of the same hand in the rectum and palpate the intervening tissue.	
POST-PROCEDURE	
Take off the gloves; look for blood on fingerstall and dispose them in 5% chlorinated solution, wash hands.	
Thank the patient and help in getting dressed.	
DOCUMENTATION	
Note the date, time and relevant information.	

Examination of Uterovaginal Prolapse 06

PREREQUISITES	
Introduce and greet the patient.	
Explain the procedure and take verbal consent.	
Reassure and instruct the patient to inform you, if she feels pain.	
Ensure patient's privacy.	
Components of examination trolley	
Appropriate light.	
Couch.	
Two draw sheets (Size: 1'x4' and 2'x4').	
Sterile gloves.	
Savlon swabs.	
Two single blade Sim's speculum.	
Cusco's speculum.	
Glass slide, ayres spatula and fixative.	
Sponge holding forceps.	
Tenaculum forceps.	
POSITION	
Expose the patient under cover of draw sheets.	
Examine in left lateral position of the patient.	
Lower leg should be straight and the upper legs flexed.	
Adjust light and wear gloves.	
PROCEDURE	
If prolapse is lying outside the introitus, assess its degree and take a pap smear.	
Manually reduce the prolapse.	

Insert Sim's speculum to retract posterior vaginal wall.	
Ask the patient to cough to demonstrate enterocele.	
If prolapse is not lying outside pull it gently with tenaculum and take a pap smear.	
Examination in dorsal position of the patient	
Help turn the patient to dorsal position. Make sure that patient remains covered properly.	
Ask patient to cough to demonstrate for stress incontinence.	
Take Pap smear if not already done.	
Pass a Cusco's speculum and take a pap smear.	
Do a bimanual examination.	
POST-PROCEDURE	
Turn off the light.	
Thank the patient and help in getting dressed.	
DOCUMENTATION	
Note the date, time and relevant information.	

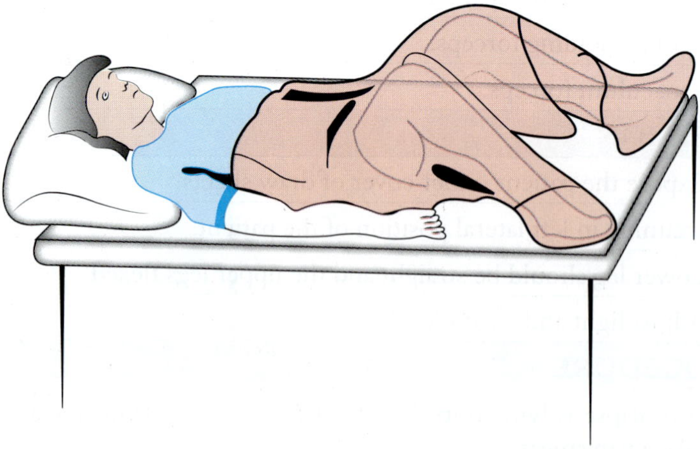

Fig. 6.1 Dorsal position

Note

For examination of uterovaginal prolapse, both left lateral and dorsal examinations are essential.

It depends on the comfort of the doctor, whether, she/he wants to start the examination in left lateral or dorsal position.

The purpose of examination for prolapse is to get complete information about the degree of prolapse cystocoele, rectocoele, enterocele and the size of uterus and palpation of adnexae.

Reference

Shaw's Obstetrics and Gynaecology

07 Pap Smear

PREREQUISITES	
Explain the procedure and the need for Pap smear.	
Take informed consent from the patient.	
Check for examination trolley.	
Instruct the patient to empty the urinary bladder.	
POSITION	
Ask the patient to undress and lie in supine position with legs abducted and flexion at the knees and should be under cover of sheet. *	
Adjust the light.	
Label the slides with marker.	
Wash or clean hands with sterillium.	
PROCEDURE	
Wear examination gloves.	
Insert the Cusco's speculum and adjust it so that the cervix is visualized.	
Take sample from whole transformation zone by rotating the Ayre's spatula at 360°.	
Quickly spread the specimen on a labelled glass slide.	
Fix the smear immediately by fixative (95% alcohol) solution or spray. The spray fixative nozzle should be held approximately 9–12 inches from the slide.	
ONE OR TWO SLIDES	
If two slides are made and placed into the same container of alcohol, the slides should be placed back to back or separated by a slide holder.	

★ Lithotomy position is not required for Pap smear or IUCD insertion.

VAULT SMEAR	
In a patient with a previous history of treatment for vaginal intraepithelial neoplasia or after hysterectomy for cervical disease, a moistened cotton swab or Ayre's spatula should be used to sample the vault and this should immediately be applied to a single slide.	
POST PROCEDURE	
Take off the gloves; dispose them in 5% chlorinated solution.	
Thank the patient and help her in getting dressed.	
Wash hands.	
Hand over the slide to the patient/appropriate person to be sent to the laboratory for cytology.	
Advise the patient to come back with result.	
DOCUMENTATION	
Date, time of procedure and relevant information.	

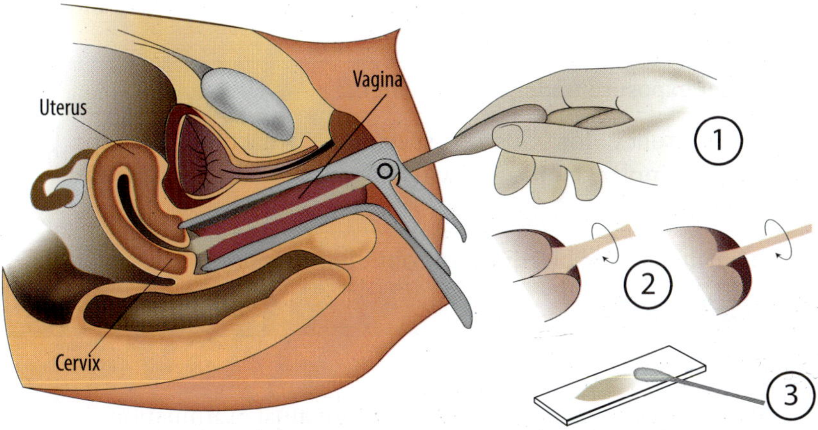

Fig. 7.1 Pap smear cytology

08 Pipelle Sampling

INDICATIONS	
Heavy menstrual bleeding.	
Post menopausal bleeding.	
Endometrial hyperplasia.	
Prior to hysterectomy.	
Evaluation of side effects of certain drugs such as Tamoxifen.	
PREREQUISITES	
Explain the procedure to the patient and reassure her.	
Take informed consent.	
Premedicate with misoprostol 200 μgm sublingually one hour and NSAID per oral 30 minutes before the procedure to prevent cramping.	
Empty the bladder.	
Ask the patient to lie in dorsal position, with legs flexed and abducted.	
Proper exposure under adequate light.	
Check trolley for Cusco's speculum, tenaculum forceps, pipelle sampler, biopsy jar with formalin, savlon swabs, and sterile gloves.	
Pregnancy, active bleeding are contraindications.	
PROCEDURE	
Wear gloves.	
Access uterine size and direction by bimanual examination.	
Introduce speculum and clean the cervix with Pyodine swab.	

Hold anterior lip of cervix with tenaculum forceps.	
Introduce uterine sound to assess size and direction of uterus.	
Introduce Pipelle according to the size of uterus.	
Create a vacuum by withdrawing the plunger.	
Perform to and fro and jiggling movements to take maximum sample from all the uterine walls.	
Remove pipelle and put the endometrial sample in formalin in the biopsy jar.	
Remove tenaculum and speculum.	
Help patient in dressing up and reassure her.	
Thank the patient.	
Label and send sample for histopathology.	
DOCUMENTATION	
Document date, time and relevant information.	
Follow up the patient with histopathology report.	

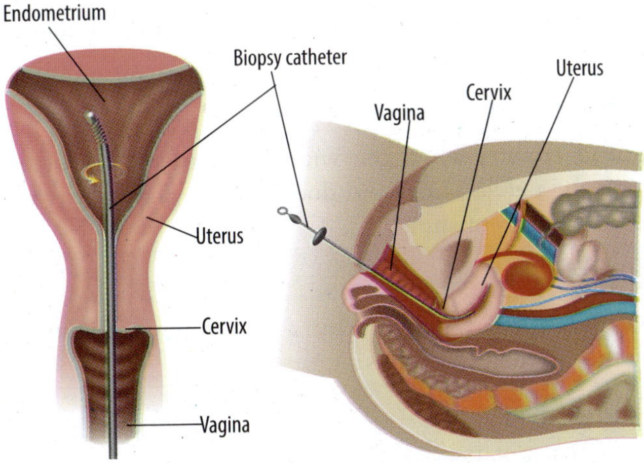

Fig. 8.1 Pipelle sampling

09 Mechanism of Labour

Mechanism of labour refers to the series of changes in position and attitude that the foetus undergoes during its passage through birth canal during labour.	
ENGAGEMENT	
Pelvis is widest in the transverse diameter at the pelvic inlet. The foetal head usually engages in the occipito–transverse position. The head is engaged when the widest part (the biparietal diameter) has passed the pelvic brim (2/5 palpable per abdomen) and zero station on pelvic examination.	
DESCENT AND FLEXION	
As labour progresses, the foetal head descends on the cervix and this flexes the head so that the vertex is leading.	
INTERNAL ROTATION	
The foetus continues to descend and on reaching the levator ani muscles, it rotates internally from occipito-transverse to occipi to-anterior position, so that the sagittal suture lies in the AP diameter of pelvic outlet.	
Further descent and crowning.	
The head crowns when the widest part of the head passes through the pelvic outlet and doesn't move backwards when the mother stops pushing.	
EXTENSION	
The well flexed head delivers by a movement of extension following the curve of the pelvis.	
RESTITUTION	
After the head has delivered, it rotates to come in line with the foetal shoulders—restitution. (The slight rotation of the occiput through 1/8 of the circle).	

EXTERNAL ROTATION	
The shoulder rotates into direct AP plane; to achieve this, occiput rotates through further 1/8 of the circle to the transverse position. This is called external rotation.	
DELIVERY OF SHOULDER AND FOETAL BODY	
When restitution and external rotation has occurred, the shoulder will be in the AP position. The anterior shoulder is under the pubic symphysis and delivers first, and the posterior shoulder delivers subsequently. Lateral traction is often exerted by gentle pulling the foetal head in the downward direction, to help release the anterior shoulder from the pubic symphysis.	
The rest of the foetal body is delivered easily, with the posterior shoulder guided over the perineum by traction in the opposite direction, so sweeping the body over the maternal abdomen.	

10 Delivery of the Placenta

IMPORTANT POINTS

Placenta should be delivered within 30 minutes of delivery of the baby.

Active or passive management to deliver the placenta.

ACTIVE MANAGEMENT

For active management of third stage of labour, five units of oxytocin are given I/V at the delivery of head in primigravida or at the time of delivery of anterior shoulder in multigravida.

Proceed to clamp and cut the cord and proceed to deliver the placenta without waiting for signs of placental separation to appear.

PASSIVE MANAGEMENT

In passive management of third stage of labour, oxytocin is not given at the time of delivery of baby.

Wait for the signs of placental separation, and then proceed to deliver the placenta.

After delivery of placenta, give five units of intravenous oxytocin.

SIGNS OF PLACENTAL SEPARATION

Lengthening of the cord protruding from the vulva.

Small gush of blood.

Fundus of the uterus becoming hard and globular and rising in the maternal abdomen.

BRANDTH ANDREW'S METHOD OR CONTROLLED CORD TRACTION FOR DELIVERY OF PLACENTA

The left hand is placed suprapubically, on the anterior surface of the uterus to elevate the fundus of the uterus.

Grasp the cord with the right hand and exert traction so that the placenta separates and is delivered.	
Delivery of the membranes follows delivery of the placenta.	
POST-PROCEDURE	
Examine the placenta for size, missing cotyledons and abruption.	
Observe for vaginal bleeding.	
DOCUMENTATION	
Active or passive management of third stage and method of delivery of placenta.	
Interval between delivery of baby and delivery of placenta.	
Delivery of complete placenta.	

11 Manual Removal of Retained Placenta

INDICATION	
Failure of placenta to deliver after 30 minutes of delivery of neonate despite active management of third stage of labour.	
Sudden haemorrhage but placenta is not delivering.	
PREREQUISITES	
Informed consent must be taken.	
Placenta should be removed manually under general anaesthesia.	
PRE PROCEDURE TASKS	
Washing up, gowning and gloving.	
Lithotomy position of the patient.	
Cleaning and draping.	
Ensuring that bladder is empty.	
PROCEDURE	
Put an extended cuff glove and arm cover on dominant hand.	
Grasp the uterus through abdominal wall, in such a manner that site of non dominant hand should be around the fundus and thumb just above pubic symphysis.	
Continue to hold the uterus stable with the non dominant hand.	
Make a cone with dominant hand (right hand for right handed people) by holding tip of fingers and thumb together, entering the vagina and gently push against cervix to enter the uterine cavity.	

Trace the umbilical cord while entering the uterine cavity, move laterally to identify the edge of placenta.	
Insert side of hand between placenta and uterine wall.	
Gently use an up and down motion to establish a cleavage plain, and then sweep behind the placenta until it is separated completely.	
Be careful not to push the tips of fingers against wall of the uterus to avoid any injury to uterine wall.	
Once the placenta is separated, deliver the placenta by the Brandth Andrew method. Sponge holding forceps may be used to hold the membranes and facilitate delivery of membranes.	
Examine the placenta and membranes to ensure completeness of the placenta and membranes. Look for missing cotyledons.	
POST PROCEDURE	
Massage the uterus to help it contract.	
Start intravenous infusion of oxytocin. Methergin may be given if not contraindicated.	
Start antibiotics.	
DOCUMENTATION	
Document the diagnosis of retained placenta in the discharge card of the patient.	
Document findings and intervention done.	
Mention about the complete delivery of placenta.	

Step 1

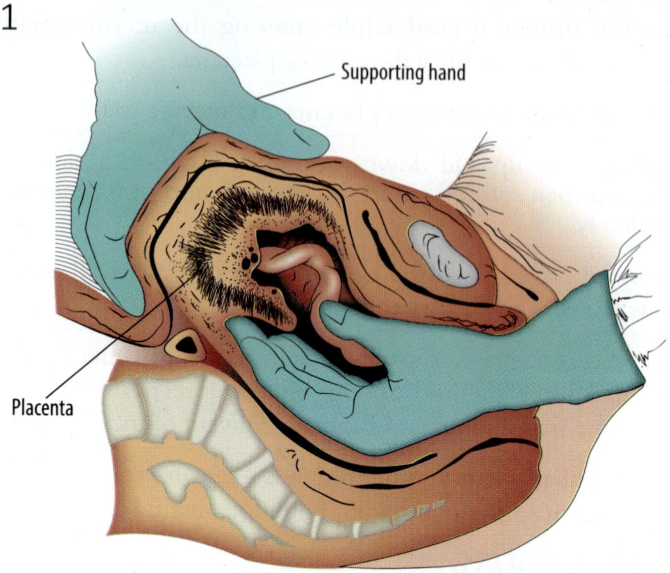

Manual removal of placenta is performed by a qualified clinician only

Step 2

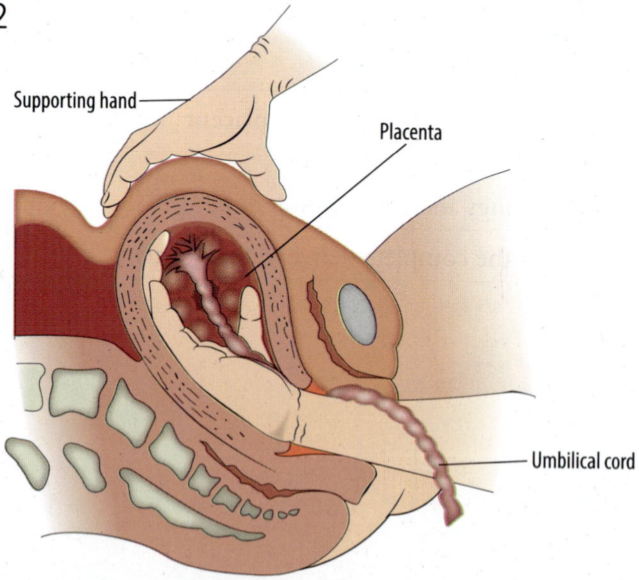

Supporting the fundus while detaching the placenta

Step 3

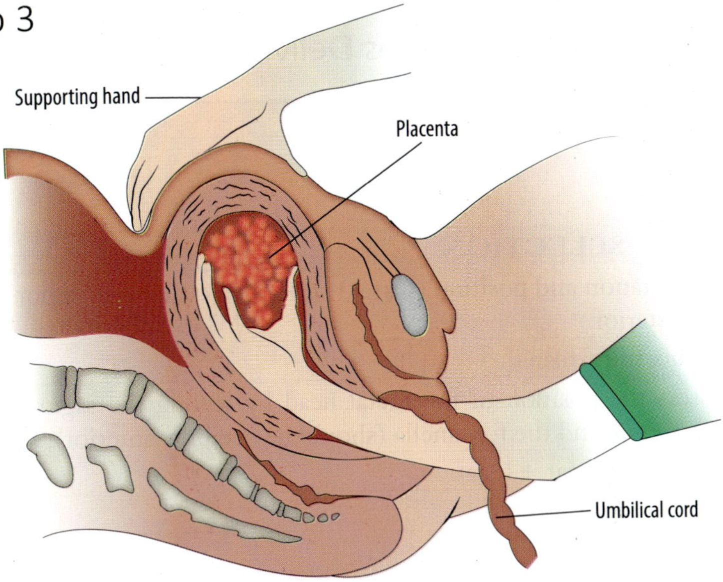

Fig. 11.1 Three steps of manual removal of placenta

12 Outlet Forceps Delivery

PATIENT SELECTION	
Presentation and position (vertex) should be occipito-anterior or posterior.	
Cervix fully dilated.	
Assess the position of the foetal head by feeling the sagittal suture line and the fontanella (should be occipito-anterior).	
Vertex at least at +1 station.	
Membranes ruptured.	
Adequate pelvis.	
PREREQUISITES	
Bladder empty.	
Adequate pain relief.	
Adequate contractions (3 in 10 minutes).	
PRE PROCEDURE TASKS	
Wash up, wear gown and gloves.	
Put the patient in lithotomy position.	
Clean the vulva with antiseptic solution.	
Drape the patient.	
Give local anaesthesia, if needed.	
PROCEDURE	
Check the pair of outlet forceps and assemble them in front of the maternal perineum with pelvis curved upwards.	
Hold left blade in left hand.	
Introduce it into the vagina in such a way that the handle lies parallel to the inguinal ligament (left side of patient).	
Use the fingers of the other hand to protect the vaginal wall from the forceps.	
Left blade once in place is handed over to the assistant.	
Apply right blade by holding forceps in right hand onto right side of the patient.	

When applied properly, the two blades should lock in such a manner that the sagittal suture runs in the centre of forceps with lambdoid suture 2 cm in front of the shank.	
After locking the forceps, apply traction in the line of pelvic axis (downwards and then forwards) synchronous with the uterine contractions and maternal expulsive efforts.	
Give sufficient support to the perineum during traction.	
Perform episiotomy at crowning (if needed).	
Between contractions, check FHR and unlock the blades.	
Discontinue the procedure, if forceps are dislodged or head fails to deliver after two tractions.	
Deliver the head of the baby and remove the forceps.	
Deliver the baby, hand over the baby to paediatrician.	
POST-PROCEDURE	
Manage third stage of the labour.	
Check the birth canal for tears and laceration and repair, if needed.	
Repair the episiotomy, if performed.	
Explain care of episiotomy and provide pain relief, if needed.	
Assessment of neonate.	
DOCUMENTATION	
Date, time, indication, and complications, if any.	

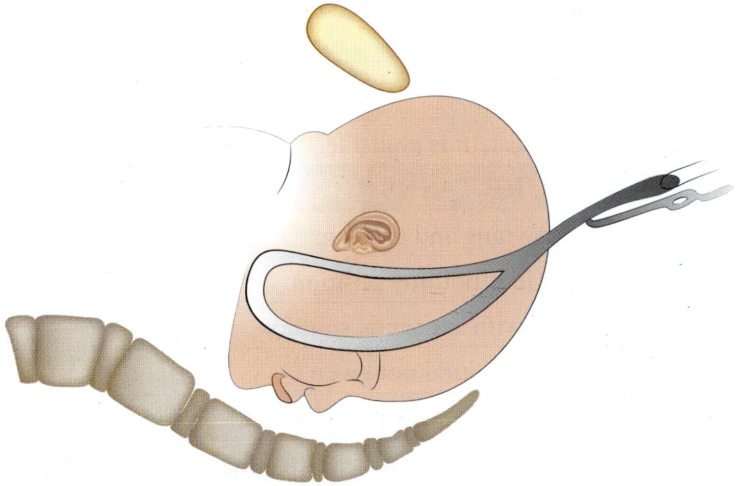

Fig. 12.1 Outlet forceps delivery

13 Vacuum Extraction

PREREQUISITES	
Obtain informed consent after explaining indications, risks, benefits and complications of procedure.	
Check the necessary equipment.	
Provide emotional support and reassurance.	
PATIENT SELECTION	
Bladder should be empty.	
Provide adequate pain relief.	
Term foetus (37 weeks beyond).	
Adequate contractions (3 in 10 minutes).	
Presentation should vertex.	
Cervix fully dilated.	
Position of the foetal head should be occipito-anterior or posterior.	
Vertex at least at +1 station.	
Membranes ruptured.	
Adequate pelvis.	
Make sure an assistant is available.	
PRE PROCEDURE TASKS	
Washing up, gowning and gloving.	
Put the patient in lithotomy position.	
Clean the vulva with antiseptic solution.	
Give analgesia if epidural not given.	
PROCEDURE	
Assess the position of foetal head (feeling the sagittal suture line and the fontanella).	

Identify the posterior fontanella.	
Apply the largest possible cup over the flexion point (3 cm) anterior to the posterior fontanella.	
Perform an episiotomy, if indicated.	
Check the application and ensure that there is no maternal tissue within the rim of the cup.	
Create a vacuum of 0.2 kg/cm² negative pressure with the pump and check the application of the cup. Increase the vacuum to 0.8 kg/cm² **OR** create a vacuum of 0.8 kg/cm² directly.	
After maximum negative pressure has been achieved, start traction in the line of pelvic axis and perpendicular to the cup along with uterine contraction.	
Between each contraction, check for: o Foetal heart rate. o Application of the cup.	
With progress, and in the absence of foetal distress, continue the guiding pulls for a maximum of 15 minutes. If the cup comes off twice during traction review and reassess indication.	
When the head has been delivered, release the vacuum by removing the tubing at the junction of the tube with vacuum machine, remove the cup and complete the birth.	
POST-PROCEDURE	
Repair the episiotomy, if performed.	
Check the birth canal for tears and laceration and repair, if required.	
Paediatric assessment of the baby.	
Explain and reassure the patient about chignon.	
DOCUMENTATION	
Date, time, indication, and complications, if any.	

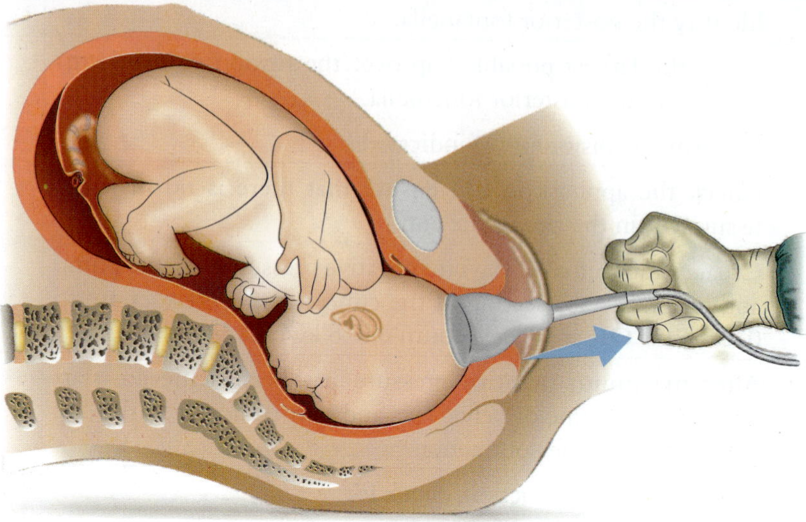

Fig. 13.1 Vacuum extraction

14 Shoulder Dystocia

Flow Chart for Shoulder Dystocia

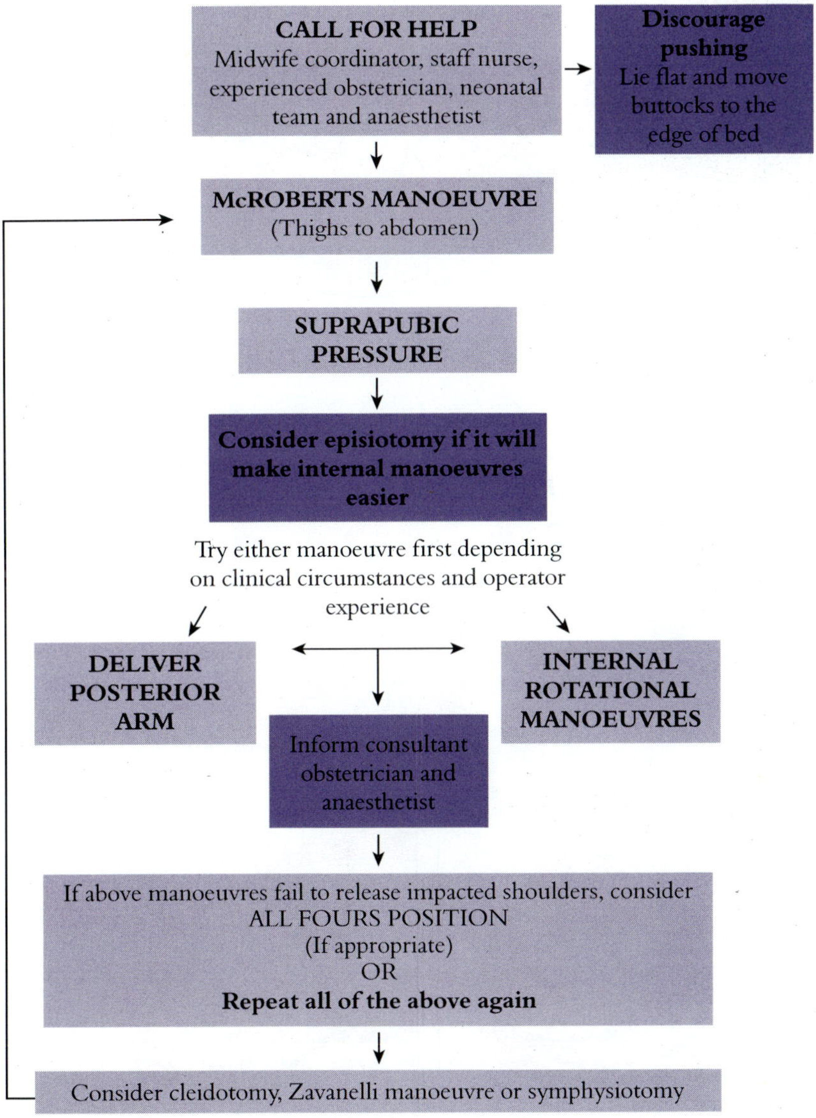

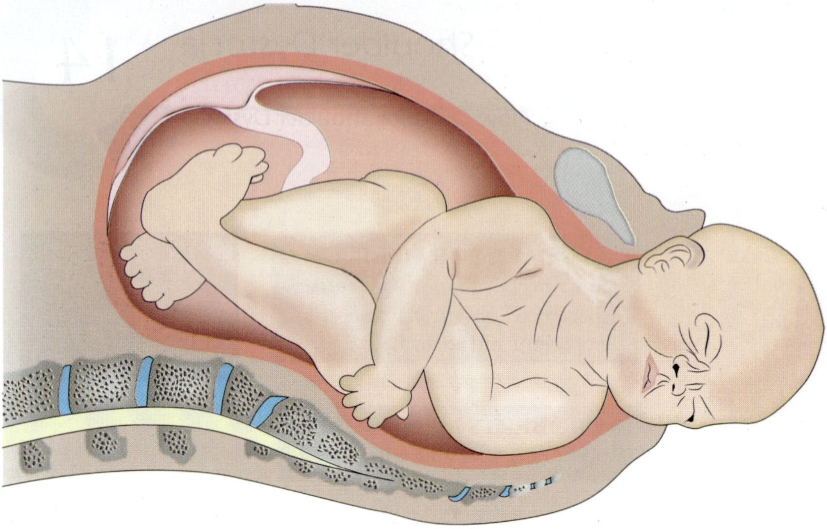

Fig. 14.1 Diagnosis of shoulder dystocia

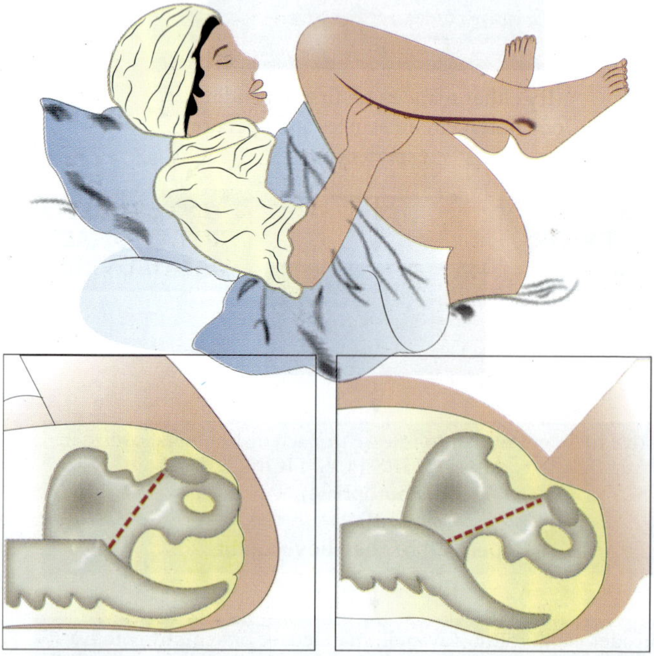

Fig. 14.2 McRoberts position

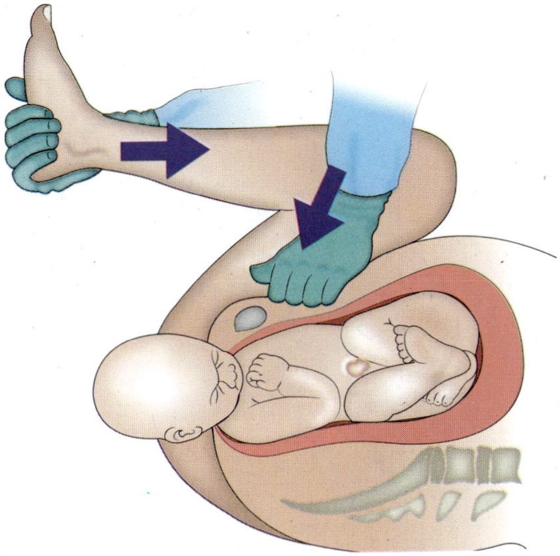

Fig. 14.3 Suprapubic pressure

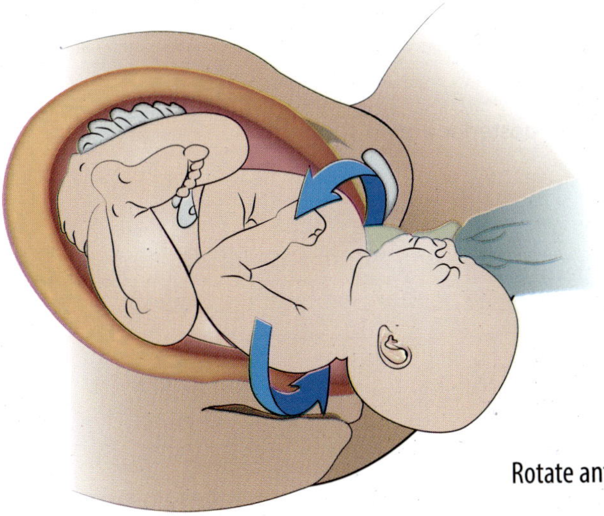

Fig. 14.4 Wood's screw manoeuvre

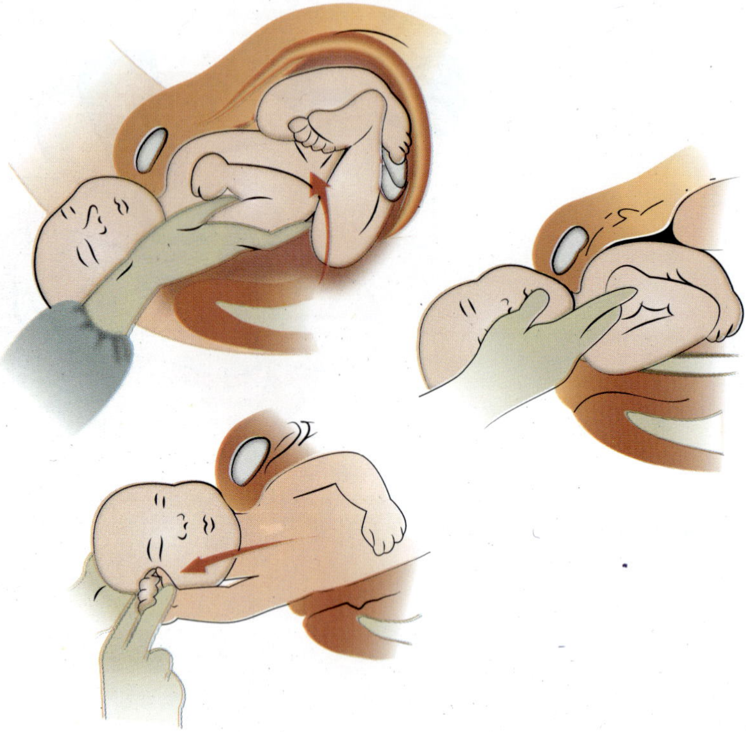

Fig. 14.5 Delivery of posterior arm

HELPERR For Shoulder Dystocia	
H	Call for help
E	Evaluate for episiotomy
L	Leg: McRoberts manoeuvre
P	External pressure–suprapubic
E	Enter: Rotational manoeuvres
R	Remove the posterior arm
R	Roll the posterior to her hands and knees

HELPERR–Pneumonic for management of Shoulder Dystocia

15 Vaginal Breech Delivery

PATIENT SELECTION	
Exclude previous C-section and/or hyper-extended neck of the foetus.	
Type of breech–extended.	
Flexed attitude of neck.	
EFW < 3.5 kg.	
Liquor adequate.	
Pelvis should be adequate.	
PREREQUISITES	
Informed consent and counselling.	
Empty bladder.	
FHR monitoring and adequate uterine contractions (3 in 10 minutes).	
IV access.	
PROCEDURE	
Hands off the breech (masterly inactivity).	
After full cervical dilatation, wait for buttocks to ascend up the perineum.	
Put patient in lithotomy position, surgeon washing up and gloving, cleaning and draping of patient.	
Analgesia: Epidural or local infiltration.	
Perform an episiotomy when the buttocks distend the perineum and fail to recede.	
Wait for spontaneous delivery of the legs.	
If legs do not deliver spontaneously, perform the Pinard's manoeuvre (abduct the thighs, flex the knee joints, and apply pressure in the popliteal fossa to deliver the legs).	

Wait for further contractions, when the umbilical cord is visible (feel pulsations) and make sure that the back of the baby is anterior.	
Release loop of cord if necessary, otherwise avoid handling.	
Drape the baby in a towel to keep it warm.	
Wait till the inferior angle of scapula is visible.	
Apply suprapubic pressure to keep neck flexed.	
Palpate for the arms in front of the chest, if flexed flip them out.	
If arms are extended deliver them by Lovset's manoeuvre (a gentle downward traction is applied and foetal trunk is rotated through 180° to deliver the arms).	
Allow descent of the head through pelvis, wait for the nape of neck to be visible at perineum (avoidance of traction will ensure the head remains fixed) and spontaneous rotation to occipitoanterior position (OA).	
Slow delivery of the head using Burns-Marshall manoeuvre (grasp the ankles with one hand and tilt the body towards mother's abdomen and deliver the head) or Mauriceau-Smellie-Veit manoeuvre (the middle finger of left hand is on the filtrum and index and ring fingers over malar eminences to promote flexion and descent of the head. The right hand is used in a similar fashion, middle finger on the nape of the neck and the index and ring finger on the foetal head to promote flexion at the neck) or by Piper's forceps.	
POST DELIVERY MANAGEMENT	
Appropriate third stage management and suturing of the episiotomy.	
Suction and neonatal support, resuscitation and assessment of neonate.	
Maintain the baby's temperature and early feeding.	
DOCUMENTATION	
Date, time, relevant information and complications, if any.	

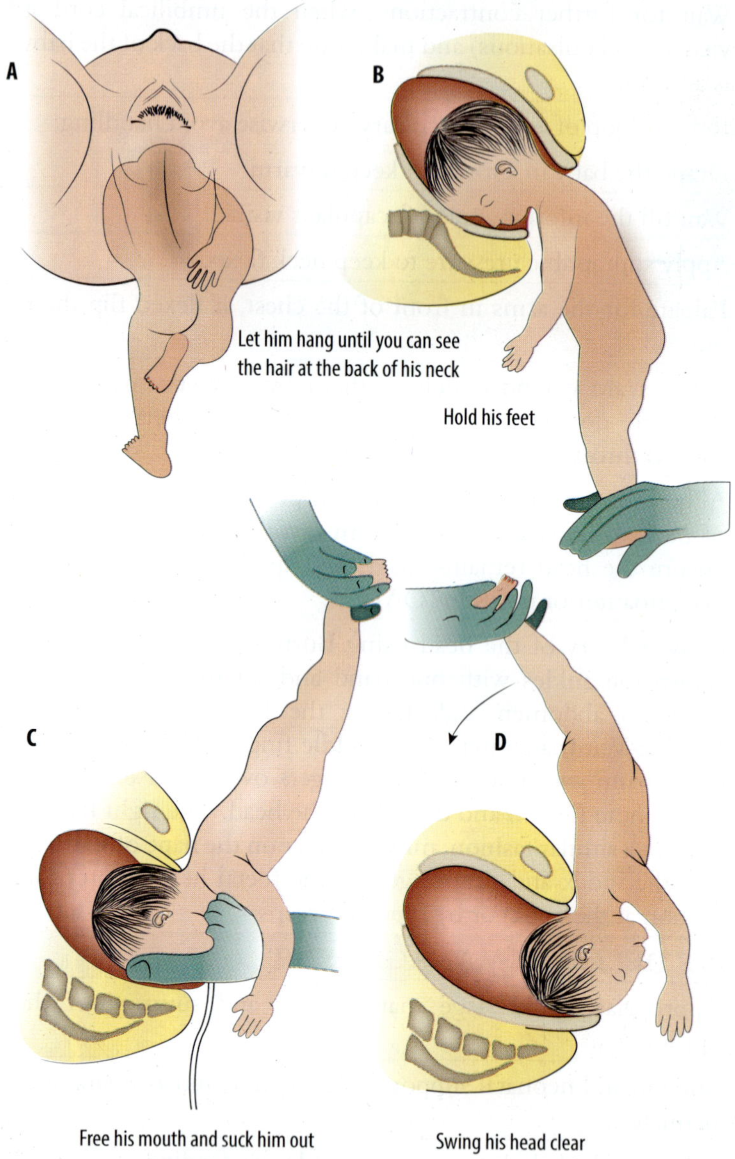

Fig. 15.1 Burns-Marshall manoeuvre

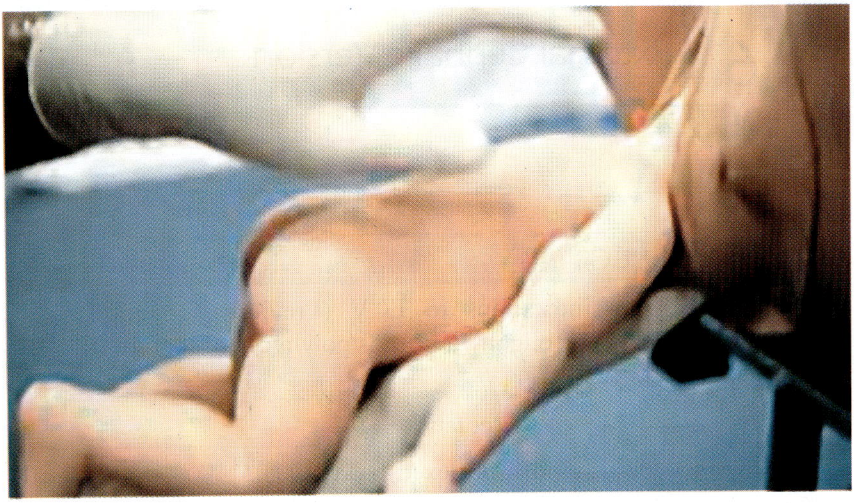

Fig. 15.2 Mauriceau-Smellie-Veit manoeuvre

16 External Cephalic Version

PATIENT SELECTION	
Rule out contraindications to ECV (Previous C-section, multiple pregnancy, oligohydramnios/polyhydramnios, foetal anomalies and IUD).	
37 weeks with breech presentation.	
Type of breech (extended or flexed) is known.	
EFW < 3.5 kg.	
Adequate liquor.	
Flexed attitude of neck.	
Pelvis should be adequate.	
PREREQUISITES	
USG for guidance.	
CTG 20 minutes trace before procedure.	
Tocolysis (Cap. Nifedipine 20 mg/oral TDS for 48 hours).	
Ask patient to empty bladder.	
Ensure I/V line.	
Analgesia if needed.	
POSITION	
Place patient in Trendelenburg position.	
PROCEDURE	
Hold the breech in right hand while left hand is placed over foetal head.	
Sustained pressure is applied by both hands simultaneously in the direction of foetal flexion for 5–10 minutes.	
Do not repeat the procedure if failed.	

POST-PROCEDURE	
Ask for abdominal pain.	
Perform USG to confirm position, FHR and CTG trace.	
Watch for PV bleeding.	
Give injection anti-D if indicated.	
Counsel and discharge the patient after two hours with advice to keep an eye on foetal movements.	
DOCUMENTATION	
Date, time, relevant information and complications, if any.	

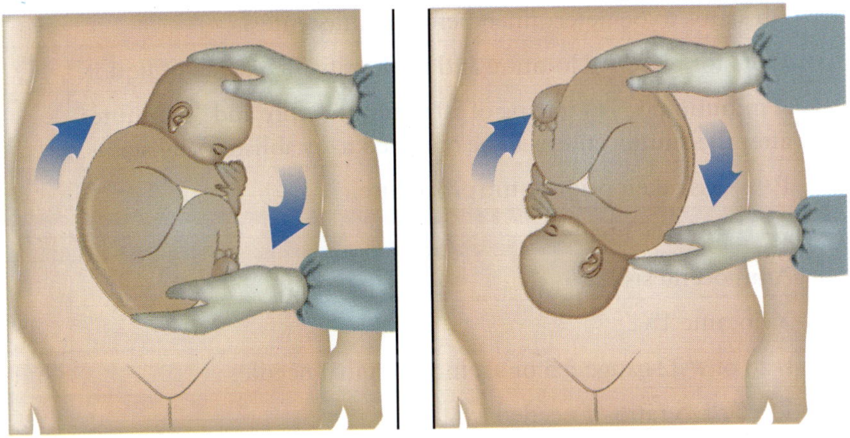

Fig. 16.1 External cephalic version

17 Amniocentesis

PREREQUISITES OF AMNIOREDUCTION	
Amniocentesis will be performed in the labour and delivery unit.	
Detailed counselling is required.	
Explain procedure to patient and take informed consent.	
Rh status to be determined before amniocentesis.	
USG for placental location and to identify the pocket of liquor.	
A minimum CTG tracing of 30 minutes before and 30 minutes after the amniocentesis to be obtained to establish foetal status.	
IV access taken prior to the procedure.	
REQUIRMENTS	
Amniocentesis kit.	
Xylocaine 1%.	
#20 or #22 gauge 3.5 or six inches spinal needle.	
Ice for L/S ratio, if needed.	
Laboratory requisition form.	
Electronic foetal monitor.	
Ultrasound.	
DRAPING	
Under aseptic measures, clean and drape the abdomen.	
PROCEDURE	
Dorsal recumbent position with wedge.	
Apply local anaesthetic prior to insertion of spinal needle.	
A 22 gauge disposable spinal needle with stillet is passed into pool of amniotic fluid under continuous ultrasound visualization, avoiding placenta and foetus.	

Stillet is removed and amniotic fluid is withdrawn with the help of syringe.	
Label the specimens with patient's name, age, registration number.	
POST-PROCEDURE STEPS	
A CTG tracing of 30 minutes should be recorded following amniocentesis.	
Patient is advised to take rest for 30 minutes and limit her physical activities for next 48 hours.	
For L/S ratio if required, place test tube on ice and transfer to laboratory.	
For genetics specimens, no ice is required. A minimum of 25 cc of amniotic fluid is required. Transfer the fluid from the syringes into the centrifuge tubes. Label the tubes with the sticker going lengthwise taking care not to cover the numbers on the tube.	
Fill out a cytogenetic requisition form which includes patient's name, age, and indication for procedure, date, time and relevant information.	
Give injection anti-D if indicated before patient is discharged.	
Provide post amniocentesis discharge instruction.	
DOCUMENTATION	
Procedure's date, time, indication and relevant information.	
Document any complications.	
FHR baseline and uterine activity should be documented both before and after the procedure on the appropriate flow sheet.	

18 Breastfeeding

EVALUATION	
History	
Comfortable nursing her baby?	
Does she rest when baby is resting (expect young baby to wake and feed during the night)?	
Is she drinking fluids (milk, juice, water) when thirsty?	
Is she eating foods from the various food groups?	
Examination	
Signs that breastfeeding is going well for mother.	
Breasts are not hard, lumpy, or tender to touch.	
Breast feels fuller before nursing her baby, and softer after nursing.	
Nipples are not sore.	
Advice	
The patient can call her doctor in case of any problem.	
POSITIONING	
Baby and mother are "tummy to tummy", when nursing the baby.	
Baby's ear, shoulder, and hip are in a straight line.	
Baby's mouth is at the nipple level while nursing.	
Support breast with thumb on top and fingers away from areola.	
LATCH ON	
Breasts get full and firm between the second and fifth day after baby's birth.	
Baby's lips are curled out (like fish lips), to get a lot of mother's areola into his/her mouth and his/her cheeks are full (not dimpled in) while nursing.	

Mother can see her baby's jaw move as she nurses.	
Mother can hear her baby sucking and swallowing on a regular basis.	
Baby should nurse as long as he wants, for about 10 to 20 minutes of active sucking and swallowing.	
ASSESSMENT OF MOTHER, BABY AND BREASTFEEDING	
Should nurse about every 1½ hours to three hours, about 8–12 times a day.	
By 4–5 days, produces about six to eight wet cloth diapers.	
Urine is clear and light yellow, not dark and orange.	
By day five, stools are soft, yellow and seedy, and occur regularly.	
During the first four weeks, has a minimum of three bowel movements a day.	
Skin is firm and healthy (not loose skin, no yellow cast).	
Face, eyes and head are full, not sunken in.	
Baby is alert and happy.	
Baby seems happy while nursing and content later.	
Baby is gaining weight.	
TEN STEPS OF BREASTFEEDING	
Follow these **ten steps** of breastfeeding based on WHO/UNICEF baby friendly hospital initiative:	
1. Have a written breastfeeding policy that is routinely communicated to all health care staff.	
2. Train all health care staff in skills necessary to implement this policy.	
3. Inform all pregnant women about the benefits and management of breastfeeding.	
4. Help mothers initiate breastfeeding within a half-hour of birth.	
5. Show mothers how to breastfeed and how to maintain lactation, even if they should be separated from their infants.	

6. Give newborns no food or drink other than breast milk unless medically indicated.	
7. Practice rooming-in—allow mothers and babies to remain together 24 hours a day.	
8. Encourage breastfeeding on demand.	
9. Give no artificial teats or pacifiers (also called dummies or soothers) to breastfeeding infants.	
10. Foster the establishment of breastfeeding support groups and refer mothers to them on discharge from the hospital or clinic.	

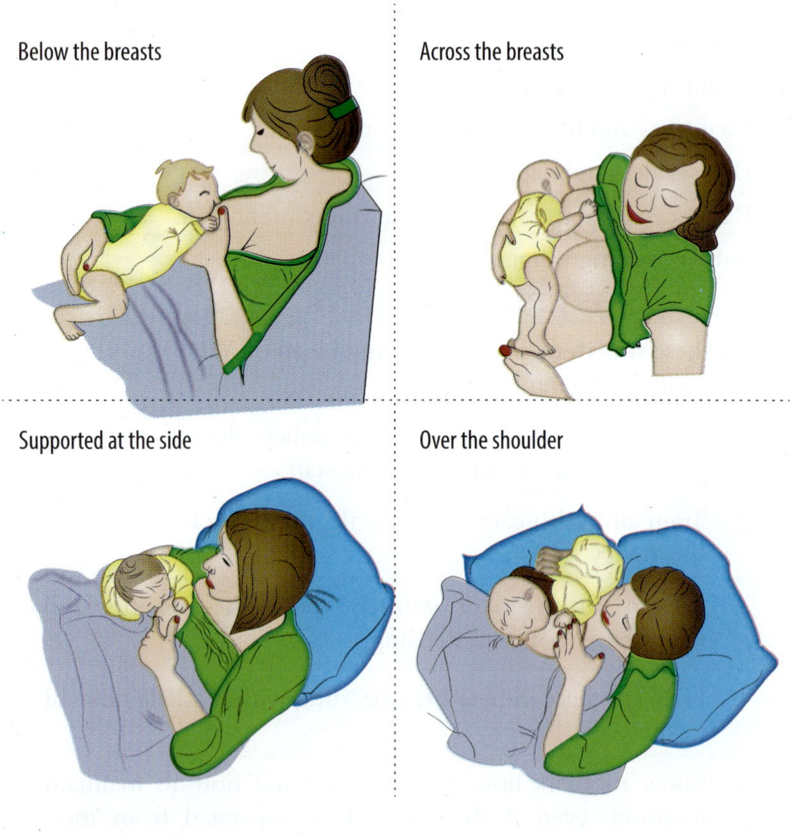

Fig. 18.1 Breastfeeding

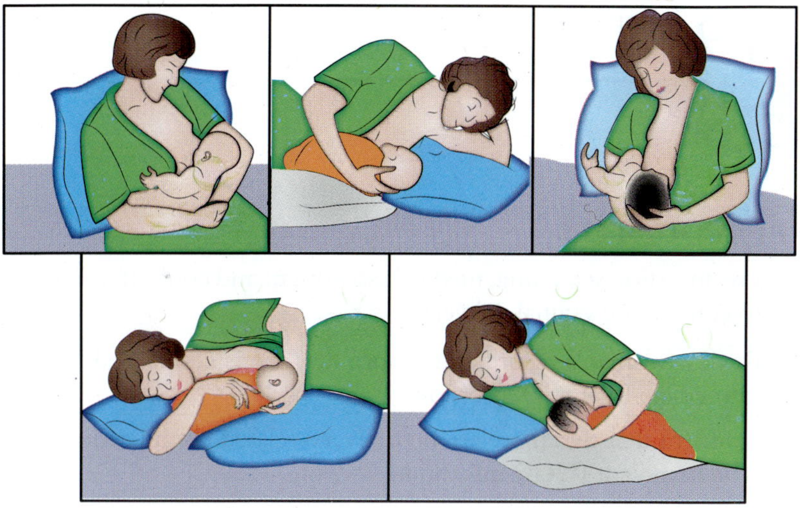

Fig. 18.2 Positions of breastfeeding

19 PPIUCD

PREREQUISITES	
Pre-insertion screening, medical assessment and consent, prior to conducting vaginal delivery. Review woman's record and ensure that she is counselled for immediate PPIUCD insertion.	
Confirm that that there are no delivery-related complications which prevent IUCD insertion. ○ Rupture of membranes for greater than 18 hours. ○ Chorioamnionitis. ○ Unresolved postpartum haemorrhage.	
If any of these conditions exist, plan re-evaluation for an IUCD at six weeks postpartum. Counsel her and offer her another method for postpartum family planning.	
Confirm that sterile instruments, supplies and light source are available for PPIUCD insertion.	
Explain the time of PPIUCD insertion and answer questions.	
PRE-INSERTION TASKS	
Arrange IUCD insertion instruments and supplies on sterile tray and wear sterilized gloves.	
Ensure active management of third stage of labour.	
Inspect perineum, labia and vaginal walls for lacerations.	
PROCEDURE	
Insertion of the IUCD	
Gently visualize cervix by depressing the posterior wall of the vagina.	
Clean cervix and vagina with antiseptic solution twice using two swabs and wait for two minutes.	

Gently grasp the anterior lip of the cervix with the ring forceps.	
Open sterile IUCD package from bottom by pulling the plastic cover, one third upwards.	
Hold IUCD package and grasp Cu-T with Kelly's placental forceps.	
Gently lift anterior lip of cervix using ring forceps and apply gentle traction to steady the cervix.	
Insert placental forceps holding IUCD into lower uterine cavity upto the point of feeling slight resistance against back wall of the uterus. Avoid touching walls of the vagina.	
Move hand to the lower part of abdomen (base of hand on lower part of uterus and fingers towards fundus) and gently push uterus upward in the abdomen to reduce the angle and curvature between the uterus and vagina.	
Gently move the placental forceps holding the IUCD upward towards the uterine fundus. Lower right hand (hand holding the placental forceps) down, to enable forceps to easily pass vaginal-uterine angle and follow the curve of the uterine cavity. Keep placental forceps closed while moving up so IUCD does not become displaced.	
Continue advancing the forceps until uterine fundus is reached.	
Open the forceps, tilt it slightly towards midline, and release IUCD at the fundus.	
Slowly remove forceps from uterine cavity, sliding instrument along the sidewall of the uterus and keeping it slightly open. Take particular care not to dislodge the IUCD or catch IUCD strings as forceps are removed.	
Stabilize the uterus until the forceps are completely out of the uterus.	
If IUCD or strings are visible protruding from the cervix, then remove IUCD, reload in sterile package and reinsert. Ensure that there is no bleeding from cervix.	
Remove all instruments used and place them in 0.5% chlorine solution in open position and ensure that they are totally submerged.	

POST-INSERTION TASKS	
Allow the woman to rest for few minutes.	
Dispose off waste material appropriately.	
Support the initiation of routine postpartum care, including immediate breastfeeding.	
Inform and assure the patient that IUCD has been successfully placed.	
DOCUMENTATION	
Document information in the patients chart or record and give her a PPIUCD card at discharge.	

Implanon 20

PRE-INSERTION TASKS	
Introduce and greet the patient.	
Check that she has been appropriately counselled and screened.	
Take informed consent.	
Discuss the insertion and removal process of IMPLANON.	
Discuss the benefits, risks and side effects. o Irregular bleeding, no bleeding, headaches, weight gain, breast symptoms. o Bruising and discomfort for up to one week after insertion. o Possibility of allergic reactions to a local anaesthetic, sex hormones, plastics, metals, latex or any other ingredients.	
Rule out pregnancy by asking for LMP.	
o Insertion at day 1–5 of menstrual cycle.	
Effectiveness of contraception at least three years.	
EQUIPMENT NEEDED	
Implanon, examination couch, sterile surgical 12x12 inch drape with hole in the centre, two mosquito forceps, small bowl, kidney tray small, sponge holding forceps and sterile gloves.	
Pyodine solution.	
Local anaesthetic plain lignocaine 1% and 2 cc disposable syringe.	
Sterile gauze, band aid and bandage.	
PROCEDURE-INSERTION	
Ask the patient to lie on her back on the examination table with the non dominant arm flexed at the elbow and externally rotated so that her wrist is parallel to her ear.	

Identify the insertion site, which is at the inner side of non-dominant upper arm about 8–10 cm (3–4–inches) above the medial epicondyle of the humerus.	
Implanon should be inserted subdermally just under the skin to avoid the large blood vessels and nerves that lie deeper in the subcutaneous tissue of the sulcus (hollow between the biceps and triceps muscles).	
Wear sterile gloves in both hands.	
Mark the insertion site with a sterile marker. Make two marks: first, mark the spot where the Implanon rod will be inserted, and second, mark a spot a few centimetres proximal to the first mark. This second mark will later serve as a direction guide during Implanon insertion.	
Clean the insertion site two times with an antiseptic solution-povidone iodine.	
Anaesthetize the insertion area by injecting 2 cc of 1% xylocaine.	
Set up the insertion kit, open and drop the applicator into the sterile area.	
Look for the Implanon rod, seen as a white cylinder at the needle's tip.	
Keeping the needle and rod sterile, remove the needle shield while holding the applicator upright.	
Apply counter-traction to the skin around the proposed insertion.	
At a slight angle (not greater than 20°), insert only the tip of the needle with the bevelled side up into insertion site.	
Lower the applicator to a horizontal position, lift the skin up with the tip of the needle, but keep the needle in the sub dermal connective tissue.	
While tenting the skin, gently insert the needle to its full length. Keep the needle parallel to the surface of the skin during insertion.	
Break the seal of the applicator by pressing the obturator support.	
Turn the obturator 90° in either direction with respect to the needle.	

While holding the obturator fixed in place of the arm fully retract the cannula.	
Confirm that Implanon has been inserted by checking the tip of needle for its absence.	
Verify the presence of Implanon in the patient's arm by palpation.	
Apply band aid over the insertion site followed by a bandage.	
POST-INSERTION TASK	
Dispose the applicator in sharp container box.	
Discuss what to do if she experiences pain, swelling, and expulsion of rods.	
Discuss the removal time of Implanon.	
Annual check up while the implant is inserted.	
DOCUMENTATION	
Document and write the insertion date.	
Provide Implanon card to the patient.	

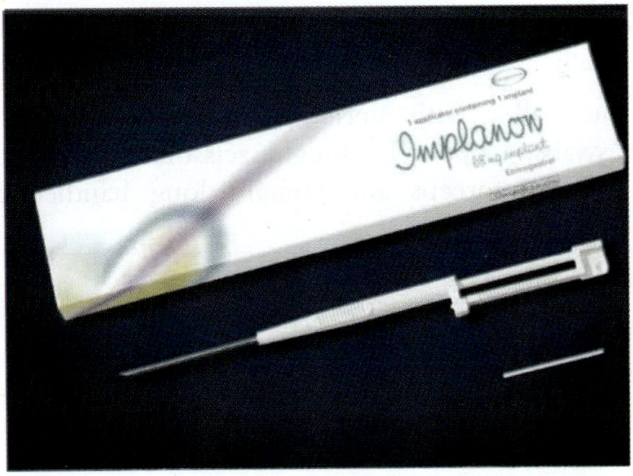

Fig. 20.1 Implanon

21 Insertion of Copper-T

PRE-INSERTION STEPS	
Counselling of the patient, regarding benefits, risks, side effects.	
Discuss insertion and removal procedures.	
Exclude pregnancy, uterine anomalies, and menorrhagia.	
Obtain consent (verbal or written).	
Premedicate with misoprostol 200 μgm sublingually one hour and NSAID orally 30 minutes before the procedure to prevent cramping.	
Perform bimanual examination to determine the position, size and direction of the uterus.	
Empty the bladder.	
Take a pap smear if indicated.	
PROCEDURE	
Insertion	
Check the trolley with sterile gloves, Cusco's speculum, Pyodine swabs, Copper-T, straight scissors, uterine sound, sponge holding forceps and straight long handled artery forceps and tenaculum.	
Wear sterile gloves.	
Perform bimanual examination.	
Insert Cusco's speculum and visualize the cervix.	
Cleanse the cervix with pyodine swab.	
Hold the anterior lip of cervix with tenaculum.	
Sound the uterus to determine its size (usually between 6–8 cm).	
Open the IUCD package and load inside the pack or outside.	

Set the upper edge of the flange to the uterine sound measurement taken previously.	
Insert the sheath along with the plunger until flange touches the cervix.	
Hold the plunger with your left hand to stabilize and then withdraw the sheath with the right hand. This will release the copper-T into the uterus.	
Gently push the plunger and sheath so that the T rests against the fundus of the uterus.	
Once IUCD is snug in the uterus, withdraw the sheath with the plunger.	
Cut the threads about 2 cm visible outside the cervix.	
POST-INSERTION STEPS	
Immediate check for vaginal spotting.	
Next visit after one month.	
Follow up visits annually if possible.	
DOCUMENTATION	
Document information in the procedure register as well as in the patient's record.	
Document any complications.	

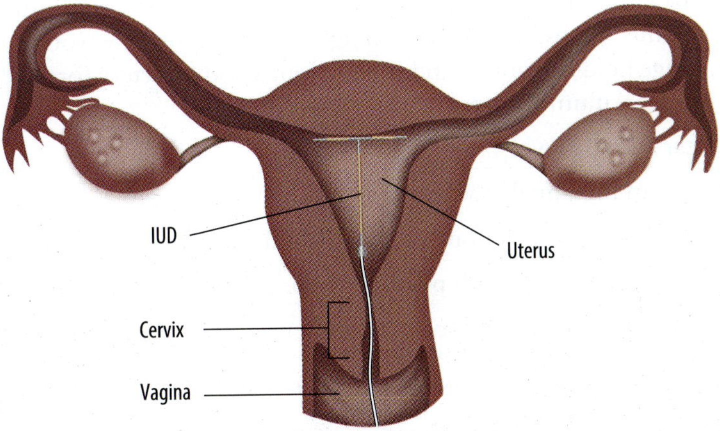

Fig. 21.1 Insertion of copper T

22 Insertion of Multiload

PRE-INSERTION STEPS	
Counselling of the patient, regarding benefits, risks, side effects.	
Discuss insertion and removal procedures.	
Exclude pregnancy, uterine anomalies, and menorrhagia.	
Obtain consent (verbal or written).	
Premedicate with misoprostol 200 μgm msublingually one hour and NSAID per oral 30 minutes before the procedure to prevent cramping.	
Perform bimanual examination to determine the position, size and direction of the uterus.	
Empty the bladder.	
Take pap smear if indicated.	
PROCEDURE	
Insertion	
Check the trolley with sterile gloves, Cusco's speculum, pyodine swabs, multiload, straight scissors, uterine sound, sponge holding forceps and straight long handled artery forceps and tenaculum forceps.	
Wear sterile gloves.	
Perform bimanual examination.	
Insert Cusco's speculum and visualize the cervix.	
Cleanse the cervix with pyodine swab.	
Hold the anterior lip of cervix with tenaculum.	
Sound the uterus to determine its size and direction.	
Open the Multiload package.	

Set the upper edge of the flange to the uterine sound measurement taken previously.	
Insert the sheath until flange touches the external OS.	
Withdraw the sheath gently. This will release the Multiload into the uterus.	
Cut the threads about 2 cm visible outside cervix.	
POST-INSERTION STEPS	
Immediate check for vaginal spotting.	
Next visit after one month.	
Follow up visits annually if possible.	
DOCUMENTATION	
Document information in the procedure register as well as in the client record.	
Document any complications.	

23 Mirena Insertion

PRE-INSERTION STEPS	
Counselling of the patient, regarding benefits, risks, side effects.	
Discuss insertion and removal procedures.	
Exclude pregnancy, uterine anomalies, fibroid distorting the endometrial cavity.	
Obtain consent (verbal or written).	
Premedicate with misoprostol 200 μgm sublingual one hour before the procedure and NSAID orally 30 minutes prior to procedure to prevent cramping.	
Perform a bimanual examination to determine position, size and direction of the uterus.	
Empty the bladder and take a pap smear, if indicated.	
INSERTION	
Check trolley with sterile gloves, Cusco's speculum, pyodine swabs, Mirena, scissors, uterine sound, sponge holding forceps and tenaculum forceps.	
Insert a Cusco's speculum, and visualize the cervix.	
Cleanse the cervix with Pyodine swab.	
Sound the uterus to determine its size (usually the size is around 6–8 cm).	
Open the Mirena package enough to reveal the shaft of the inserter.	
Wearing sterile gloves make sure that the slider is in the furthermost position away from you.	

Pull on the threads to place the system in the insertion tube and fix the threads in the cleft at the end of the shaft.	
Set the flange according to the uterine sound measurement taken previously.	
Move the plunger and sheath gently into the uterus until the flange is about 2 cm away from the cervix.	
Release the arms of the system by pulling the slider back until it reaches the raised mark on the shaft.	
Push the inserter gently inwards until the flange touches the cervix.	
Release the system completely by pulling the slider back all the way; threads will release automatically.	
Remove the system from the uterus. Cut the threads to have about 2 cm visible outside the cervix.	
POST-INSERTION STEPS	
Check for vaginal spotting.	
Next visit after one month.	
Follow up visits annually if possible.	
DOCUMENTATION	
Document information in the procedure register as well as in the patient's record.	
Document any complications.	

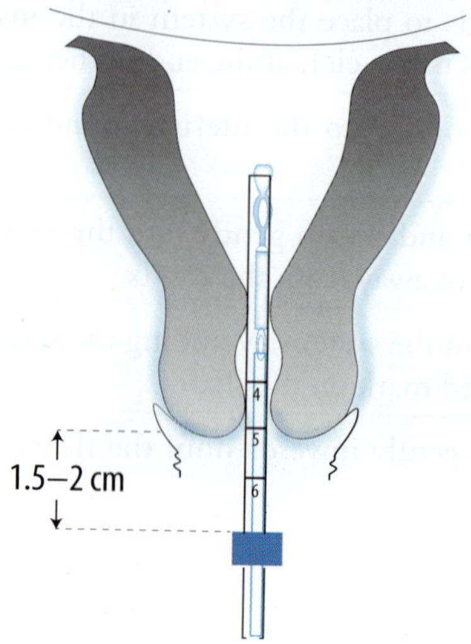

Fig. 23.1 Adjusting the flange 1.5–2/cm from the external OS

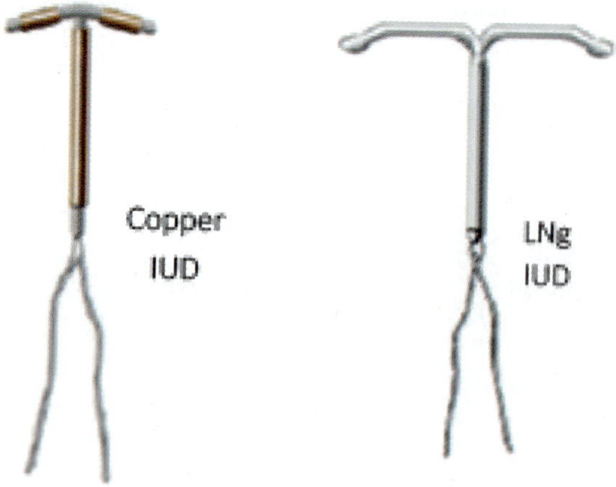

Fig. 23.2 Copper IUD and Mirena

Insertion of Foley Catheter 24

PREREQUISITES	
Patient's privacy, appropriate light and couch.	
Foley catheter of appropriate size (16 Fr.), urine bag, disposable 10 cc syringe filled with distilled water, lignocaine gel, sterile gloves, Savlon swabs.	
Counsel and explain the purpose of the procedure, if the patient is awake.	
Check trolley to ensure the availability of required supplies.	
PROCEDURE	
The patient is undressed under cover of draw sheet and put in dorsal position with legs flexed and abducted.	
Sterilized gloves of appropriate size are worn.	
The labia are parted and held between thumb and forefinger and the urinary meatus is cleaned with Savlon swab in an above downward movement and the swab is disposed off. This is repeated three consecutive times keeping labia parted at all times.	
Ask the assistant to open the external packing of the Foley catheter pack.	
Open internal packing of Foley catheter and attach urine bag to one end.	
The urine bag should be closed properly distally.	
Properly visualize the urethral opening.	
Introduce the tip of Foley catheter into urethra and push it in further, when urine starts coming out.	
Inflate the balloon of Foley catheter with 10 cc distilled water with the help of syringe.	
Make sure that balloon is inflated properly.	

Fix the catheter at the inner side of the thigh.	
Straighten the legs of patient.	
DOCUMENTATION	
Date, time and relevant information.	
Document the amount and colour of urine.	

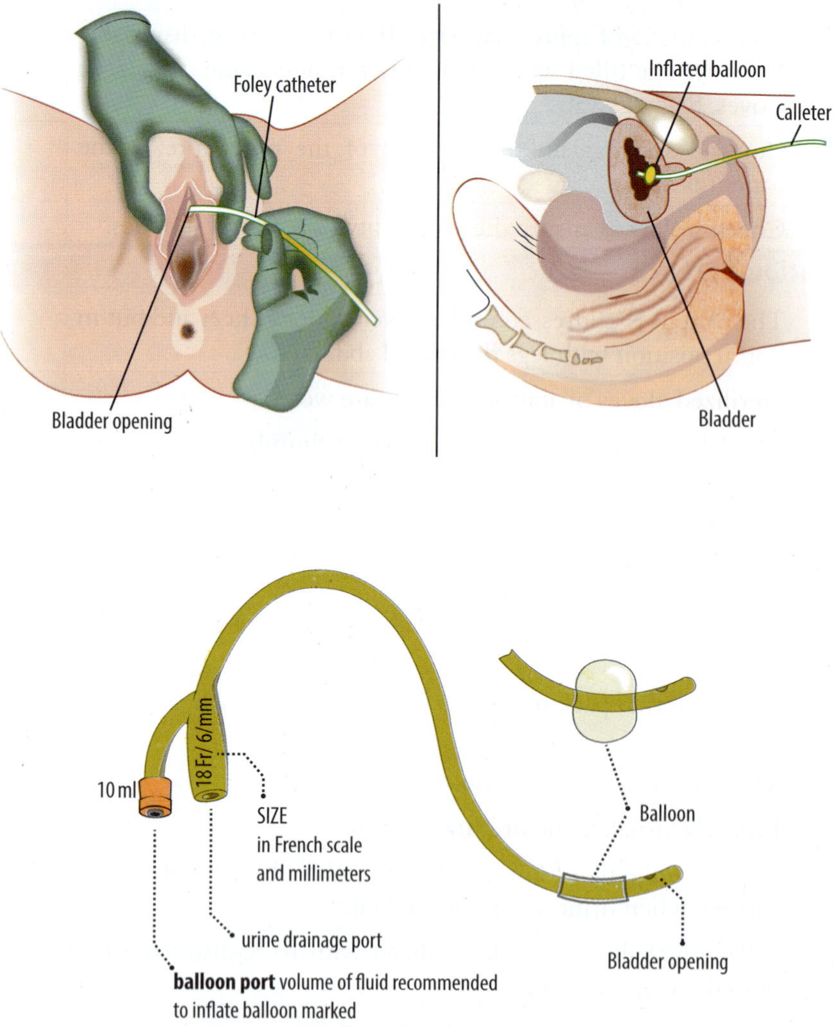

Fig. 24.1 Urinary catheterization by Foley catheter

25 Gowning and Gloving

GOWNING	
The folded gown is lifted directly upward from sterile package.	
Step back from the table into an unobstructed area.	
The neckband is located and the gown is held just below the neckband with fingertips.	
Let the gown unfold. It has to be ensured that the inside of the gown is kept towards the body without touching the sterile exterior of the gown with bare hands.	
The gown is held at the shoulder level and both arms slipped in simultaneously.	
During gowning it has to be ensured that the gown does not touch anywhere.	
The assistant ties the gown.	
GLOVING	
Closed gloving technique	
In closed glove technique, the surgeon's hands remain inside the sleeves and should not touch the cuffs.	
Both hands are kept within the cuffs.	
The folded cuff of the left glove is grasped with the right hand.	
The palm of glove is placed against the palm of left hand (the glove fingers point up the forearm).	
The glove is pulled over the extended fingers onto the wrist by pushing the hand through the glove until it completely covers the cuff of the glove.	

The right hand is gloved in the same manner by reversing the above steps.	
The gloves are checked for integrity after completion of gloving.	
Open gloving technique	
In the open glove technique the surgeon's hands slide all the way through the sleeves out beyond the cuff.	
The sterile glove of the left hand is lifted and hand inserted into the glove and pulled upon. The cuff remains folded till the other glove is donned and only then it will be pulled upon to complete the gloving process. Bare hand does not touch the outside of the glove.	
Wear the right glove in similar fashion.	
Assisted gloving	
Palm of the glove is held towards the surgeon.	
The cuff is stretched to open the glove.	
The other hand is gloved in a similar fashion.	

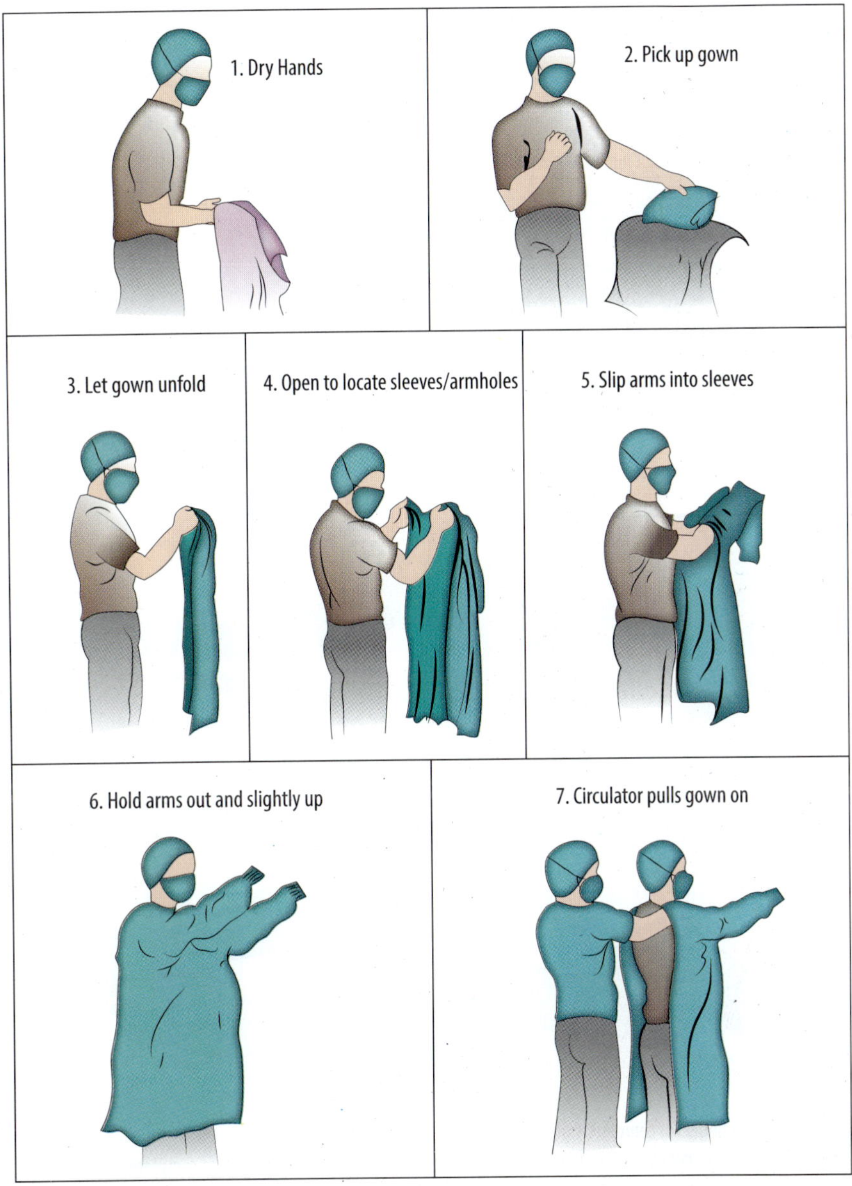

Fig. 25.1 Gowning

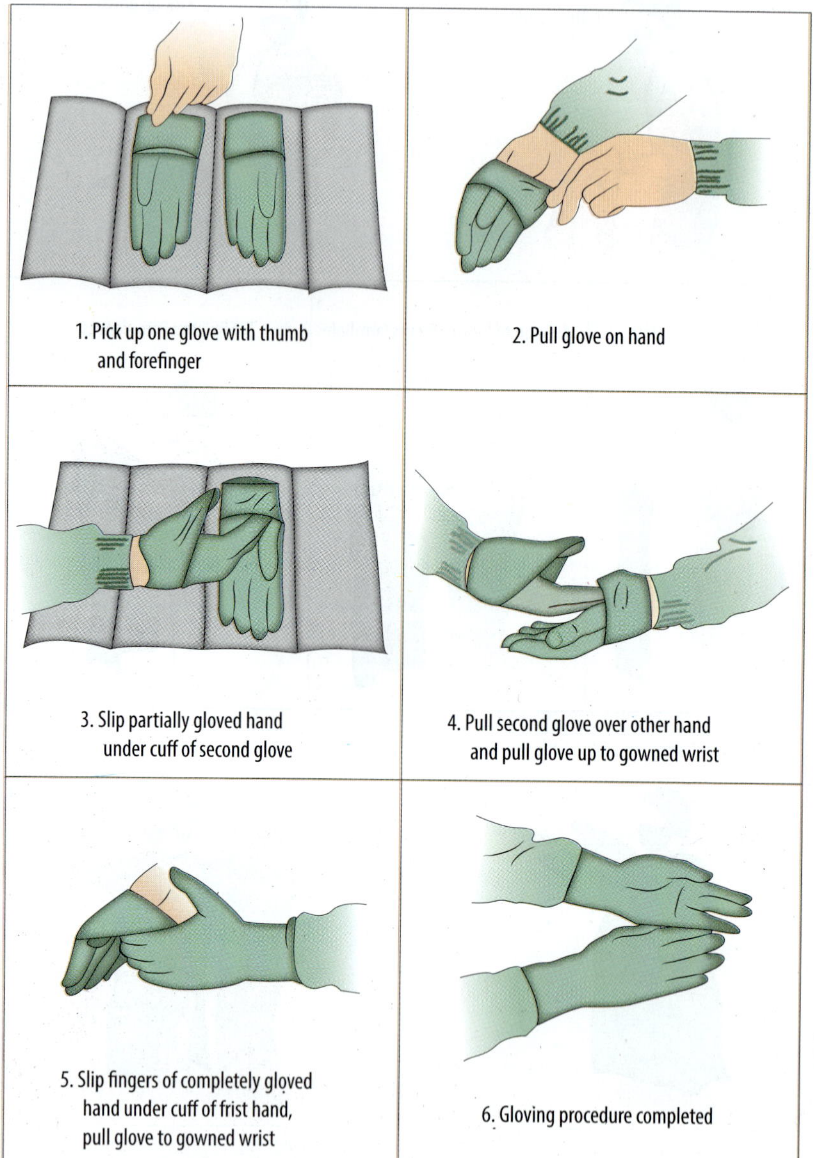

Fig. 25.2 Gloving

26 Opening of Abdomen

PREREQUISITES	
Aseptic measures should be ensured.	
Comfortable position of surgeon with proper adjustment of operative table.	
Good light.	
PROCEDURE	
Pfannenstiel incision is a transverse abdominal incision 2 cm above pubic symphysis approximately 10–12 cm long, slightly convex towards the pubis though length is adjusted according to need of procedure.	
The fat is incised down to the rectus sheath and aponeurosis of external oblique muscle.	
Small vessels in the fat are tied or cauterized.	
Two small incisions are given on either side of midline in the rectus sheath.	
The short incisions in the rectus sheath are now extended for the full length of the skin incision using curved scissors.	
The upper and lower edges of the incision are grasped with four Allis forceps on either side of the midline and the underlying muscle is separated from the sheath by combination of blunt (swab) and sharp dissection (straight scissors or diathermy).	
Small vessels running parallel to midline are cauterized or tied.	
Rectus muscle is now separated with two fingers vertically or in previous surgery by scissors. Avoid cutting the rectus muscle.	
The parietal peritoneum is held with two artery forceps as high as possible to avoid injury to the urinary bladder.	
Avoid holding the intestine in the artery forceps while opening the peritoneum.	

A small incision is given by a scalpel between the two artery forceps to open the peritoneum. While opening the peritoneum, ensure that there is no injury to the intestine.	
Extend the peritoneal incision upward and downward, avoiding injury to the urinary bladder.	
DOCUMENTATION	
Document date, time and procedure.	

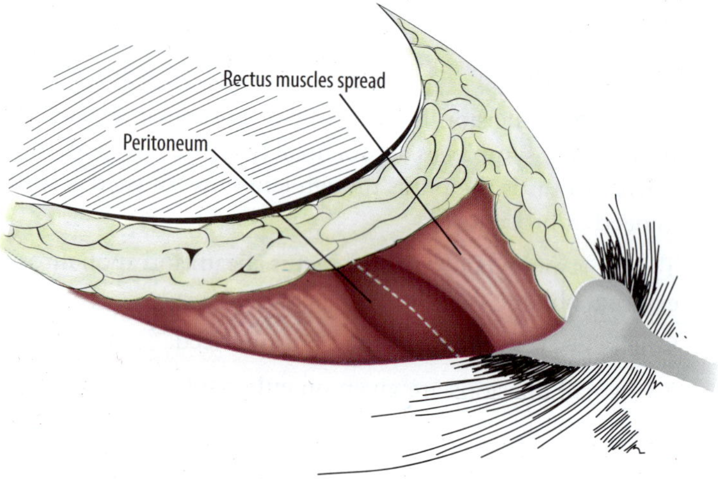

Fig. 26.1 Opening of abdomen

Balloon Tamponade 27

The principal of balloon tamponade is exerting a tamponade effect on the uterine walls to stop bleeding in non traumatic PPH.	
INDICATIONS	
PPH, when pharmacological measures fail to control PPH.	
CONTRAINDICATIONS	
Fibroid or any congenital anomaly of uterus causing distortion of uterine cavity.	
Purulent infection of vagina and cervix.	
Allergy to balloon material (silicon, rubber)	
Suspected uterine rupture.	
PREREQUISITES	
Informed consent.	
Lithotomy position.	
Bladder should be empty, insert Foley catheter if not already placed.	
Coagulopathy should be ruled out.	
THINGS REQUIRED	
Foley catheter 16FR.	
Condom (condom tied with the black silk to the Foley catheter 3–4 cm away from the tip of catheter, not so tight).	
Silk No.1	
50 cc bladder wash syringe.	
Normal saline 1000 cc.	
USG machine.	
Good light source.	
PROCEDURES	
Aseptic measures.	
Take 16FR Foley catheter fitted with condom.	

Tie its lower end with Silk no. 1	
50 cc bladder wash syringe.	
Retract posterior vaginal wall with Sims retractor.	
Hold anterior lip of cervix with sponge holding forceps.	
Insert catheter fitted with condom inside the uterine cavity. Taking it to the fundus of the uterus preferably under USG guidance.	
Inflate with 250–500 ml normal saline with the help of bladder syringe and ligate the lower end of catheter to prevent back flow after filling the condom.	
Leave in situ for 24–48 hours.	
POST PROCEDURE	
Monitor BP pulse, temperature, fundal height and per vaginal bleeding.	
Watch for PV bleeding.	
Reverse coagulopathies, if any.	
Bladder should be continuously drained.	
Starts antibiotics.	
Oxytocin infusion for 24 hours.	
Mention amount of fluid filled.	
REMOVAL OF CATHETER	
Leave balloon tamponade in place for 24 hours.	
Withdraw half of the normal saline, if no significant bleeding after 30 minutes, withdraw the remaining volume to deflate and remove the balloon.	
Continue to observe patient for any active bleeding.	
DOCUMENTATION	
Date and time of procedure.	
Document volume of normal saline infused.	
Document estimated blood lose.	

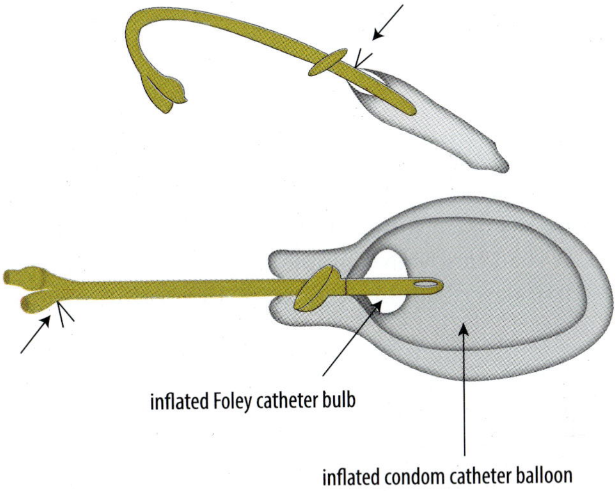

Fig. 27.1 Balloon tamponade

28 B-Lynch Suture

DEFINITION	
B-Lynch suture is a brace suture applied to atonic uterus in case of severe PPH. It is an innovative simple fertility and uterus sparing technique. First described in 1997 by **Christopher Balogun Lynch.**	
INDICATIONS	
Uterine atony.	
Massive bleeding after mid-trimester miscarriages.	
Prophylactically in patients with high risk of PPH where no facility for blood transfusion.	
CONTRAINDICATIONS	
Fibroid uterus.	
DIC.	
Arterial bleeding requiring exploration and ligation.	
COMPLICATIONS	
Hematometra.	
Pyometra.	
Asherman's syndrome.	
Localized area of uterine necrosis.	
PREREQUISITES	
Control of bleeding with manual compression of uterus, assessment of the bleeding should be done by the visual inspection.	
PROCEDURE	
Open abdomen in layers.	
Exteriorize the uterus and open the uterus through previous scar.	

Check the efficacy of B-Lynch suture by compressing the uterus between the palms of both hands.	
Suture used is chromic catgut #2 on 70 mm needle or Vicryl number 1 suture.	
Start applying the suture from 3 cm before the lower edge of incision 3 cm medial to lateral border of right side of uterus and come out 3 cm above the upper edge of incision 4 cm medial to lateral border on right side.	
Cross over the fundus and pass the suture (at the level of anterior incision) on right side from posterior uterine wall into uterine cavity and come out of uterine cavity in posterior uterine wall on left side at the same level.	
Again cross over the fundus on left side. Repeat the suture anteriorly on left side as on right side.	
Tie the knot anteriorly below the uterine scar and close the uterine scar in layers.	
Replace the uterus into abdominal cavity.	
Check for per vaginal bleeding.	
Close abdomen in the reverse order after securing haemostasis.	
POST-PROCEDURE	
Monitor pulse, BP, PV bleeding, fundal height half hourly for four hours then one hourly for four hours.	
Continue oxytocin infusion for 12–24 hours.	
Give antibiotics.	
Build up Hb by blood transfusion if required.	
DOCUMENTATION	
Document time and date of procedure.	
Document indications, detail of procedure, intra-operative findings and post procedure orders.	

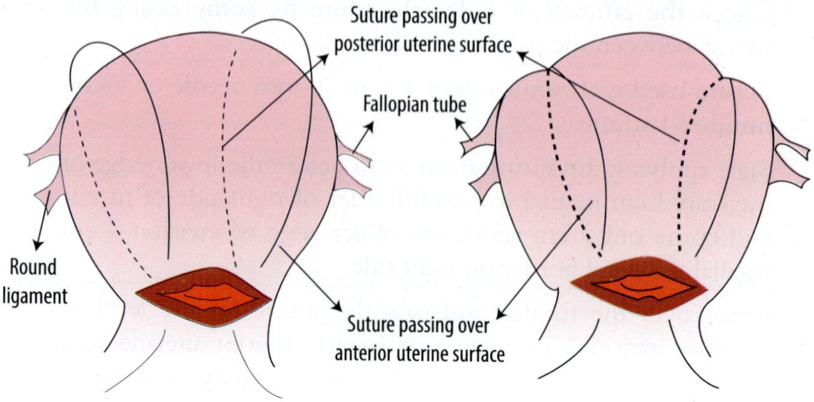

Fig. 28.1 Steps of B-Lynch suture

SECTION 02

GENERAL PROTOCOLS

Introduction to General Protocols

Protocols provide recommendations to trainees and practitioners on delivering high quality, appropriate care to patients with specific clinical conditions or diseases. It details the outline of the steps to be followed in the treatment of a patient. The protocols are short, easy to apply and can be used as a tool to monitor the quality of patient care.

29 Hyperemesis Gravidarum

DESIRED PATIENT OUTCOMES	
Patient should maintain pregnancy with minimal complications.	
Patient should experience improvement with no significant weight loss.	
After management, patient should not require parenteral nutrition.	
Capacity building of patients to use family support and counseling.	
CRITERIA FOR WARD ADMISSION	
Significantly abnormal urea and electrolytes (sodium > 120 mmol/l).	
Loss of 10% body weight.	
Haematemesis.	
Severe abdominal pain or symptoms suggestive of another cause for vomiting.	
Persistent vomiting after day case rehydration.	
Persistent large ketosis on urinalysis after day case rehydration.	
Three previous attendances for day case rehydration.	
CLINICAL ASSESSMENT AND CARE	
Confirmation of foetal heart beat by ultrasound.	
Assess nausea and vomiting, its triggers, causes, duration and frequency.	
Assess and record patient baseline weight and vital signs.	
Baseline investigations (CBC, blood group, BSR, hepatitis serology, urine C/E).	

Send specific investigations—serum electrolytes, blood urea level, liver function tests and obstetrical ultrasound.	
Implement dietary consults.	
Monitor intake and output.	
Monitor frequency and volume of emesis.	
Dietary supplements, enteral or parenteral nutrition for 24–48 hours if needed.	
Psychological support, possibly psychiatric consult, if need be.	
Encourage spouse and family members to become involved with patient care.	
Interventions to improve oral tolerance: ○ Eat small frequent meals with low fat protein. ○ Drink fewer liquids with meals. ○ Avoid foods like fatty, greasy, fried, spicy, very sweet or having strong odours. ○ Eat easily digested starches, like rice, potatoes, noodles, cereal and bread. ○ When feeling nauseated, slowly sip on carbonated beverages.	
Vitamin/mineral supplements. ○ Tablet pyridoxine or doxylamine 10 mg orally at bed time.	
Antiemetic drugs. ○ Promethazine 12.5–25 mg I/V or orally every four hours. ○ Prochlorperazine 25 mg directly every 12 hours. ○ Ondansetron, pregnancy category B drug belongs to a class of medications called serotonin $5HT_3$ receptor antagonists.	
Dosage: 4–8 mg orally or 10 mg I/V eight hourly can be used for refractory class of hyperemesis not controlled with other medication.	
Motility agents. Metoclopramide 5–10 mg 6–8 hours orally, intramuscular or intravenously.	

Antihistamine medications. ○ Meclizine 25–50 mg orally every 12–24 hours. ○ Dimenhydrinate 50–100 mg orally every 4–6 hours. ○ Diphenhydramine 25–50 mg orally/IM/IV every 4–8 hours.	
Corticosteroid. Methylprednisolone 16 mg orally or IV every eight hours for three days tapered over two weeks in cases of improvement (best avoided before 10 weeks of gestation).	
Electrolyte and fluid replacement.	
INSTRUCTIONS AT TIME OF DISCHARGE	
Report to the hospital in case of worsening nausea, vomiting, or abdominal pain.	
Decrease in weight from baseline weight.	
DOCUMENTATION	
Document assessment findings and interventions.	
Document patient response to care in patient's progress notes.	

Reference:

ACOG Recommendations April 2013 and Medscape

Precipitate Delivery Management in Labour Ward

30

POLICY
First Stage
All labour rooms will have a bulb sucker and cord clamp in a prominent location.
A precipitate delivery kit containing appropriate emergency equipment (i.e. clamps, scissors, and bulb sucker) is readily available in the labour ward at all times.
CLINICAL ASSESSMENT AND CARE
It is necessary to make rapid assessment of the patient.
Provide support to the perineum to minimize trauma.
Assist patient with delivery of presenting part. If umbilical cord is around neck, gently slip it off. Assist patient with remainder of delivery.
When the baby is delivered, clamp umbilical cord approximately three inches from baby's abdomen with plastic clamp and cut between with sterile scissors. Use bulb sucker to keep baby's airway patent.
Wrap the baby and hand it over to the paediatrician.
Notify the paediatrician about patient's history, gestational age, any maternal medications and any meconium noted.
Examine for vulva vaginal laceration.
Monitor patient's vital signs and vaginal bleeding.
Administer medications and/or transfer patient to delivery area.
DOCUMENTATION
Document the procedure.
Record time of delivery of infant and placenta.

31 Postpartum Care in Hospital—12 Hours

OBJECTIVES	
Patient should demonstrate no signs of postpartum complications.	
Patient should receive an acceptable level of pain relief.	
CLINICAL ASSESSMENT AND CARE	
Assess vital signs, pain relief, assess fundal height, ensure contraction of the uterus and watch for the excessive vaginal bleeding and perineum (including episiotomy, haemorrhoids) at least every 30 minutes for two hours, then every eight hours until discharge.	
Administer analgesics as needed.	
Give Anti-D immunoglobulin, if indicated.	
After epidural analgesia, assess sensation and movement of lower limbs and dressing site.	
Assess IV line for function.	
Assess status of bladder by observing displacement of fundus both before and after voiding. Continue assessment until patient has two spontaneous voids > 200 cc (catheterize if unable to void six hours post-delivery).	
Examine breast and encourage early feeding.	
INSTRUCTIONS	
Maternal-infant attachment and bonding at the time of delivery.	
Ensure early breastfeeding.	
Assist in first ambulation.	
Assist care of baby until mother is alert.	
Instruct patient to report pain or heavy vaginal bleeding.	

Regular diet with increased fibre and plenty of fluid.	
Stool softener or laxative.	
Instruct about immunization of the baby.	
Counselling of patient for warning signs and immediate reporting to hospital if they arise.	
Instruct patient for infant's security.	
INSTRUCTIONS	
Follow up after ten days in vaginal delivery, three weeks in caesarean section and visit at six weeks for both.	
DOCUMENTATION	
Document the time and mode of delivery.	
Document postpartum complications, if any.	

PROTOCOLS

FOR DRUGS

Prostaglandin E_2 Vaginal Tablet (3 mg) 32

POLICY	
Indications for induction of labour should be clearly documented.	
According to ACOG recommendations, the practice of an elective induction without a valid indication is not recommended.	
DESIRED PATIENT OUTCOMES	
Patient will show evidence of cervical ripening by improvement in Bishop score.	
Patient should be free of complications.	
CLINICAL ASSESSMENT AND CARE	
Confirm gestational age, lie, presentation, and indication for induction of labour.	
Rule out contraindications to vaginal delivery (Cephalopelvic disproportion, placenta praevia, vasa praevia, cord prolapse, prior uterine surgery).	
Confirm lie of foetus, presenting part, its position and station in pelvis.	
FHR tracing for at least 20 minutes.	
Perform Bishop score.	
PROCEDURE	
Prostaglandin E2 vaginal tablet (3 mg) is placed in the posterior fornix of the vagina.	
Patient to remain recumbent for at least 30 minutes.	
Maintain patent IV access.	
Uterine contractions usually are evident in the first hour and exhibit peak activity in the first four hours. Uterine hyperstimulation can occur as late as nine hours after placement.	

Patient is allowed clear liquids orally.	
Reassess the patient after six hours and repeat the dose, if needed.	
Reassess the patient after six hours of the second dose.	
Generally prostaglandin E_2 vaginal tablet (3 mg), two doses are recommended but for the third dose, decision has to be made at consultant level.	
REPORTABLE CONDITIONS	
Uterine hyperactivity.	
Any non-reassuring foetal heart rate pattern.	
Vaginal bleeding.	
Ruptured membranes.	
DOCUMENTATION	
Document the procedure.	
Induction delivery interval.	
Document the doses of Prostaglandin E_2 vaginal tablet (3 mg).	
Maternal outcome (SVD or C/S).	
Foetal outcome.	

References:

RCOG Guidelines, 2012

33 Misoprostol

(Preinduction Cervical Ripening and Induction of Labour)

POLICY	
Indication for induction of labour should be clearly documented.	
Misoprostol is contraindicated in patient with previous caesarean section.	
According to ACOG recommendation, an elective delivery prior to 39 weeks without a valid indication is not recommended.	
DESIRED PATIENT OUTCOMES	
Patient will show evidence of cervical ripening by improvement in Bishop score.	
Patient should be free of complications.	
CLINICAL ASSESSMENT AND CARE	
Confirm gestational age, lie, presentation, and indication for induction of labour.	
Rule out contraindications to vaginal delivery.	
Confirm lie of foetus, presenting part, its position and station in pelvis.	
FHR monitoring and Bishop scoring.	
Misoprostol is contraindicated in patients with previous caesarean section.	
PROCEDURE	
20 minutes CTG trace prior to cervical ripening.	
Obtain vital signs and maintain I/V access.	
Advise patient to remain recumbent for at least 30 minutes after vaginal dose.	
25 μg vaginally four hourly (maximum six doses) or 20 μg oral solution two hourly (maximum 12 doses) for oral solution, dissolve 200 μg of misoprostol tablet in 200 ml of water in a container.	

Uterine contractions usually are evident in the first hour and exhibit peak activity in the first four hours. Uterine hypersitumulation can occur as late as 10 hours after placement.	
Patient is allowed clear liquids orally.	
Reassess the patient after four hours and repeat the dose if needed.	
Oxytocin if indicated should be started six hours after the last Misoprostol.	
REPORTABLE CONDITIONS	
Uterine hyperactivity.	
Any non-reassuring foetal heart rate pattern.	
Vaginal bleeding.	
Ruptured membranes.	
DOCUMENTATION	
Time and date of induction.	
Induction delivery interval.	
Complications.	
Mode of delivery.	
Foetal outcome.	
Patient should be free of complications.	

References:

FIGO Guidelines, 2012

34 Oxytocin Infusion

PURPOSE	
To administer oxytocin in a safe and controlled manner.	
POLICY	
Oxytocin for the purpose of induction or augmentation of labour.	
Oxytocin administration should be performed only in labour room.	
The practice of elective delivery prior to 39 weeks gestation is best avoided.	
PRE-REQUISITE	
Rule out contraindications to vaginal delivery (complete placenta previa, vasa previa, cord prolapse, foetal malposition and CPD).	
Suitable vertex presentation and favorable cervix.	
CTG trace of 20 minutes prior to induction and then two hours after induction.	
Cervical ripening should be done in patients with poor Bishop score.	
PROCEDURE	
Select dose in milliunits/min.	
Enter the volume to be infused.	
Begin oxytocin infusion at five milliunits/min and increase by five milliunits/min every 30 minutes (in case of primigravida, at 10 unit of oxytocin in 1000 ml of Ringer's Lactate and in case of multigravida add five unit of oxytocin to 1000 ml of Ringer's Lactate. In case of cardiac patient, add five unit of oxytocin to 500 ml of Ringer's Lactate).	

If 10 IU of oxytocin are added in 1000 ml Ringer's Lactate then 1 ml of Ringer's Lactate would contain 10 milliunits of oxytocin.	
1 ml of Ringer's Lactate or 10 milliunits of oxytocin is equal to 16 drops/min of infusion and five milliunits of oxytocin is equal to eight drops/min of infusion.	
Starting dose: Start at five milliunits/min of infusion which is equal to eight drops/min and then increase the infusion every 30 minutes by eight drops/minute to a maximum dose of 51 drops per min which is equal to 32 milliunits/min of infusion.	
Monitor. ○ Uterine contractions (Three contractions in 10 minutes). ○ Foetal heart rate after every 30 minutes in first stage and every five minutes in second stage of labour.	
Decrease oxytocin: ○ If there are more than three contractions during 10 minutes. ○ The uterine resting tone is increased. ○ Abnormal foetal heart rate tracing.	
Discontinue if: ○ Uterine hypersitumulation. ○ Foetal distress.	
Restarting oxytocin: a If discontinued< 30 minutes. ○ Uterine hyperstimulation: Oxytocin 4 milliunits/min lower than the previous level. ○ Foetal indications: Restart oxytocin at 2/milliunits/min. b If the oxytocin discontinued >30 minutes, restart at 2/ milliunits/min.	
DOCUMENTATION:	
Note the date, time, dose of oxytocin and relevant information.	

Severe Pre-Eclampsia/Eclampsia 35

DESIRED PATIENT OUTCOMES

Patient should be delivered at an appropriate time safely.

Patient and foetus should have minimal complications during the delivery process.

Make appropriate referrals to support services as indicated.

CLINICAL ASSESSMENT AND CARE

Assess maternal BP on admission, every 15 minutes until patient is stabilized, then every 30 minutes in initial phase of assessment, then four hourly if patient is stable and asymptomatic.

Pulse, respiration, and FHR on admission, then at least every eight hours or more often.

Urinary proteins daily.

Danger signs	
Headaches, dizziness	Oedema, reflexes, clonus, convulsions
Visual changes (blurring of vision, diplopia)	Proteinuria (> 0.3 g in 24 hours)
Epigastric pain/vomiting	Abnormal liver enzymes (ALT or AST > 70 IU/L)

LABOUR AND DELIVERY ROOM CLINICAL CARE

Place patient in left lateral position.

Apply external foetal monitor.

Vital signs every 1–2 hours, more often if necessary.

Check reflexes and clonus every two hours.

CONTROL SEIZURES

Begin **Magnesium Sulphate**.

Obtain baseline vital signs and FHR tracing.

Check deep tendon reflexes, and vital signs prior to administration and document.

Create a treatment kit (MgSO4, I/V fluids, I/V sets, urine bag, Foley catheter, blood collection vial, lignocaine 2% solution, calcium gluconate1 g (10 ml of 10% solution).

Route	Loading dose	Maintenance dose
I/V	4 g MgSO4 20% by infusion pump over 5–10 minutes	1 g/hour for 24 hours after last fit. Add 12 g (24 ml) of 50% $MgSO_4$ in 76 ml of normal saline @ 8 μ drops/min
I/M	10 g of 50% MgSO4 solution, 5 g in each buttock, as deep IM injection with 1 ml of 2% xylocaine in the same syringe.	5 g I/M in alternate buttock every four hour for 24 hours after delivery or the last convulsion.

Recurrent seizures

Should be treated with either a future bolus of 2 g magnesium sulphate or an increase in the infusion rate to 1.5 to 2 g/hour.

Monitor: urine output (>30 ml/hour), respiratory rate, oxygen saturation, patellar reflex every 15 minutes for first two hours and then every 30 minutes.

Continuous foetal monitoring during magnesium sulfate therapy.

Reassess vital signs at the end of the loading dose and at least every 2 hours during magnesium sulfate therapy.

Send investigations. CBC, blood group Rh-factor, urine C/E, LFTs, RFTs, serum uric acid, clotting profile if platelet <100x106/L.

Check serum magnesium level daily if continue for > (therapeutic range 4–7Eq/L).

Maintain intake and output during administration.

Stop therapy: If urine output is <20 ml/hour, patellar reflexes are absent, respiratory rate is <16/min, oxygen saturation is <90%.

Antidote: 10% calcium gluconate, 10 ml I/V over 10 minutes.

CONTROL HYPERTENSION

Consider **labetalol** for BP>160–170 mmHg systolic or >100–110 mmHg diastolic.

ORAL

An initial 200 mg oral dose, check BP after 30 minutes, repeat the dose if needed within one hour.

INTERMITTENT BOLUS IV ADMINISTRATION

Indication; If there is no response to oral treatment.

Co-administer labetalol 200 mg or 20 mg nifedipine while gaining I/V access.

Give preload of 250 ml of N/Saline 0.9% or Hartmann's immediately before use.

Label syringe with "labetalol 100 mg in 20 ml".

Inject 20 mg (4 ml) over two minutes.

The maximum labetalol bolus dose rate is 50 mg/minute(max effect five minutes).

Monitor BP and HR every five minutes until stable.

If no change, repeat labetalol 20 mg (4 ml) every 10 minutes (titrated to BP) to a maximum of four doses (80 mg = 16 ml) .

Once stabilised, monitor BP every hour for four hours then return to preeclampsia regimen.

INTRAVENOUS LABETALOL INFUSION

If the BP is not controlled after 4 I/V bolus doses:

Syringe driver	Infusion pump
Set up: Draw up labetalol 200 mg (40 ml) undiluted. Write "labetalol 5 mg/ml" and attach label to syringe.	**Set up:** Add 200 mg labetalol (40 ml) to 60 ml of NaCl 0.9%. Label "labetalol 2 mg/ml in NaCl 0.9% (labetalol 200 mg/100 ml)

Syringe driver infusion dose	Infusion pump dose
Start infusion at 4 ml/hour (20 mg/hour). Titrate to stabilise blood pressure by adjusting every 30 minutes to a maximum of 32 ml/hour (160 mg/hour). Discontinue by weaning over 1–2 hours when BP is < 155/95 mmHg.	Start infusion at 10 ml/hour (20 mg/hour). Titrate to stabilise blood pressure by adjusting the infusion as required every 30 minutes to a maximum dose of 80 ml/hour (160 mg/hour). Discontinue by weaning over 1–2 hours when BP is < 155/95 mmHg.

Control level obtained:

- Monitor BP and HR every hour for up to 6–8 hours after the last dose of labetalol.
- Maintain patient in the left lateral position, on strict bedrest.
- Continuous foetal heart rate monitoring.
- Cardiac monitoring should be considered in cardiac patients.
- **Hydralazine** can be used for the acute management of severe hypertension.
- 5–10 mg I/V undiluted pushed over two minutes.
- If BP is still excessive after 20 minutes, administer 10 mg IV push over two minutes.
- After 20 minutes if blood pressure is still high, monitor blood pressure and heart rate every five minutes for 20 minutes.
- Once BP is achieved, repeat BP every 10 minutes for one hour, then every 15 minutes for one hour, then every 30 minutes for one hour, the every four hours.

PLANNING DELIVERY

Foetus < 34 weeks

Delivery can be deferred, Dexamethasone 12 mg, two doses, 12 or 24 hours apart, given I/M. The benefits of conservative management should be reassessed after 24 hours.

Foetus > 34 weeks

Once assessment is done, plan delivery

- Patients with eclampsia should be delivered within 12 hours of the fit.
- Severe pre-eclampsia should be delivered within 24 hours of diagnosis.
- If vaginal delivery is possible, it is usually safer for the patient.
- C-section should be done for malpresentation, foetal distress, failure to progress.
- Misoprostol, prostaglandins or a Foley can be used for cervical ripening.
- If patient has C-section watch for coagulopathy.
- General anaesthesia is generally preferred and ketamine should not be used.

POSTPARTUM

Continue $MgSO_4$ until 24 hours after delivery or continue until 24 hours after last fit.

Continue antihypertensive therapy as long as BP is over 110 diastolic.

Monitor urine output.

HELLP syndrome—consider steroid therapy.

Monitor for oliguria more than 48 hours after delivery.

Monitor for coma lasting more than 24 hours after the last fit.

DOCUMENTATION

Treatment given, complications and relevant information should be documented.

References

RCOG Guidelines, 2006

36 Hydralazine

(Pregnancy Induced Hypertension)

POLICY	
External foetal monitoring should be done.	
Monitoring of blood pressure is mandatory.	
Maternal cardiac monitoring may be neede donly in cardiac patients.	
DESIRED PATIENT OUTCOMES	
Maintain blood pressure140/90 in order to maintain utero placental perfusion.	
Prevention of maternal and foetal complication associated with severe hypertension.	
Optimal maternal and foetal well-being with minimal side effects.	
CLINCIAL ASSESSMENT AND CARE	
Care of the patient: ○ Hydralazine should be considered for blood pressures systolic ≥160 or diastolic ≥110. ○ Obtain baseline vital signs prior to the administration of hydralazine. ○ Keep patient in lateral position.	
Administration: ○ 5–10 mg I/V undiluted pushed over two minutes. ○ If BP is still excessive after 20 minutes, administer 10 mg IV pushed over two minutes. ○ After 20 minutes if blood pressure is still high, monitor blood pressure and heart rate every five minutes for 20 minutes. ○ Once normal blood pressure is achieved, repeat blood pressure, every 10 minutes for one hour, then every 15 minutes for one hour, then every 30 minutes for one hour, then every four hours.	

PATIENT TEACHING	
Instruct patient to report any side effects experienced. ○ Dizziness or lightheadedness. ○ Nausea or vomiting.	
WARNING SIGNS	
Increase in blood pressure.	
Change in foetal heart rate baseline or variability.	
Inability to control blood pressure at maximum dose of hydralazine.	
Difficulty breathing, shortness of breath and/or chest pain.	
Tachycardia, hypotension.	
Dizziness, lightheadedness, headache, any neurologic changes.	
Nausea and vomiting.	
DOCUMENTATION	
Vital signs.	
Foetal heart rate and uterine activity.	
Rate changes in blood pressure with continuous hydralazine infusion.	
Side effects of therapy.	

Reference:

RCOG Guideline 2006

37 Labetalol

(Hypertensive Disorders of Pregnancy)

DESIRED PATIENT OUTCOMES

Control of the patient's blood pressure in order to maintain uteroplacental perfusion.

CLINICAL ASSESSMENT AND CARE

Obtain vital signs prior to the administration.

Consider Labetalol for BP>160–170 mmHg systolic or >100–110 mmHg diastolic.

ADMINISTRATION OF LABETALOL

Oral

An initial 200 mg oral dose, check BP after 30 minutes, repeat the dose if needed within an hour.

Intermittent Bolus IV Administration

Indication; If there is no response to oral treatment.

Co-administer Labetalol 200 mg or 20 mg Nifedipine while gaining I/V access.

Give preload of 250 ml of N/Saline 0.9% or Hartmann's immediately before use.

Label syringe with "Labetalol 100 mg in 20 ml".

Inject 20 mg (4 ml) over two minutes.

The maximum Labetalol bolus dose rate is 50 mg/minute(max effect five minutes)

Monitor BP and HR every five minutes until stable.

If no change, repeat Labetalol 20 mg (4 ml) every 10 minutes (titrated to BP) to a maximum of four doses (80 mg = 16 ml) .

Once stabilised, monitor BP every hour for four hours then return to preeclampsia regimen.

Intravenous labetalol infusion

If the BP is not controlled after four I/V bolus doses:

Syringe driver	Infusion pump
Set up Draw up Labetalol 200 mg (40 ml) undiluted Write "Labetalol 5 mg/ml" and label the syringe	**Set up** Add 200 mg Labetalol (40 ml) to 60 ml of NaCl 0.9%. Label "Labetalol 2 mg/ml in NaCl 0.9% (Labetalol 200 mg/100 ml)
Syringe driver infusion dose Start infusion at 4 ml/hour (20 mg/hour). Titrate to stabilise blood pressure by adjusting every 30 minutes to a maximum of 32 ml/hour (160 mg/hour). Discontinue by weaning over 1–2 hours when blood pressure is <155/95 mmHg.	**Infusion pump dose** Start infusion at 10 ml/hour (20 mg/hour). Titrate to stabilise blood pressure by adjusting the infusion as required every 30 minutes to a maximum dose of 80 ml/hour (160 mg/hour). Discontinue by weaning over 1–2 hours when blood pressure is <155/95 mmHg.

CONTROL LEVEL OBTAINED

Monitor blood pressure and heart rate every hour for up to 6–8 hours after the last dose of labetalol.

Maintain patient in the left lateral position, on strict bed rest.

Continuous foetal heart rate monitoring.

Cardiac monitoring should be considered in cardiac patients.

REPORTABLE CONDITIONS

BP< 140 mmHg systolic, HR<60/minute.	Change in foetal heart rate.
Difficult breathing, wheezing, bronchospasm.	Dizziness, headache, nausea, vomiting

DOCUMENTATION

Vital signs, foetal heart rate and uterine activity.

Rate changes to continuous labetalol infusion.

Side effects of therapy.

References:

1. The Confidential Enquiry into Maternal and Child Health (CEMACH) 2007.
2. Australian Product Prescription Guide (APPG).
3. (RCOG). The management of severe pre-eclampsia/eclampsia. Guideline No. 10A March 2006.

38 Magnesium Sulfate

(Use in Hypertensive Disorders of Pregnancy)

PURPOSE

To delineate care of the patient receiving magnesium sulfate.

SUPPORTIVE DATA

Magnesium sulfate is therapy of choice for the prevention and control of seizures in hypertensive disorders of pregnancy.

DESIRED PATIENT OUTCOMES

Prevention and control of seizures with minimal side effects.

PATIENT INSTRUCTIONS

Discuss commonly experienced side effects and symptoms of toxicity and its treatment with the patient, if any that may be used.

Explain the plan of care during magnesium sulfate therapy, i.e., frequent vital signs, checking deep tendon reflexes.

Instruct patient to call the doctor if she has difficulty breathing or is short of breath at any time during magnesium sulfate therapy.

Procedure (administration of magnesium sulfate)

Obtain baseline vital signs.

Assess foetal heart rate tracing for baseline and long-term variability.

Obtain deep tendon reflexes prior to administration and with each set of vital signs.

Create a treatment kit (MgSO4, I/V fluids, I/V sets, urine bag, Foley catheter, blood collection vials, lignocaine 2% solution, calcium gluconate1 g (10 ml of 10% solution).

Begin magnesium sulfate:

Route	Loading dose	Maintenance dose
I/V	4 g (8 ml) $MgSO_4$ in 96 ml of N/S 20% by infusion pump over 5–10 minutes	1 g/hour for 24 hours after last fit.Add 12 g (24 ml) of 50% $MgSO_4$ in 76 ml of normal saline @ 8 μ drops/min
I/M	10 g of 50% $MgSO_4$ solution, 5 g in each buttock, as deep IM injection with 1 ml of 2% xylocaine in the same syringe.	5 g I/M in alternate buttock every four hours for 24 hours after delivery or the last convulsion.

Recurrent seizures

Further bolus of 2 g magnesium sulphate or an increase in the infusion rate to 1.5 to 2 g/hour.

Monitor: Urine output (>30 ml/hour), respiratory rate, oxygen saturation, patellar reflex every 15 minutes for first two hours and then every 30 minutes.

Continuous foetal heart monitoring during magnesium sulfate therapy.

Vital signs at the end of the loading dose and every two hours during $MgSO_4$ therapy.

Send investigations: CBC, blood group, Rh-factor, urine C/E, LFTs, RFTs, serum uric acid, clotting profile if platelet <100x106/L.

Check serum magnesium level daily if continue for >24 hours (therapeutic range 4–7 Eq/L).

Maintain intake and output during administration.

Stop Therapy: If patellar reflexes absent (first sign), urine output is <20 ml/hour, respiratory rate is <16/min, oxygen saturation is < 90%.

WARNING SIGNS

Absent reflexes	Abnormal lab values
Shortness of breath or chest pain.	Deep sedation—patient difficult to arouse.

DOCUMENTATION

Document vital signs, reflexes, and side effects of therapy.

Reference:

RCOG Guideline 2006

39 Nifedipine

Administration for Tocolysis

POLICY	
Initiation of oral Nifedipine loading doses should be administered only in labour room due to the need for close maternal and foetal monitoring.	
Compared with beta agonist, Nifedipine is associated with improvement in neonatal outcome, although there is no long term date.	
DESIRED PATIENT OUTCOMES	
Patient should be counseled about the understanding of premature labour and foetal risks associated with premature delivery.	
Patient should be counseled regarding the goals of Nifedipine therapy.	
Patient should have cessation of uterine activity for maintenance of the pregnancy.	
Patient should have minimal or no complications as a result of Nifedipine therapy.	
Counselling regarding the signs and symptoms of premature labour.	
PROCEDURE	
Begin electronic foetal monitoring and obtain a baseline for 20 minutes.	
Monitor patient's BP, pulse, foetal heart rate every 15 minutes in first hour and then half hourly.	
Daily uterine contraction monitoring (minimum of 30 minutes) should be done to assess uterine status.	
Explain procedure and side effects to the patient.	

Potential side effects may include: Hypotension, headache, nausea, tachycardia, facial flushing, dizziness, chest pain, nasal congestion, heartburn and neuromuscular blockade (in combination with magnesium therapy).	
INITIAL DOSE OF NIFEDIPINE	
Optimal dose in preterm labour is yet to be determined. However in most studies the initial dose was 20 mg orally or sublingually. If contractions persisted, this dose was repeated over 15–20 minutes upto a maximum of total dose of 40 mg during the first hour of treatment. Then 20 mg orally every 6–8 hours for 2–3 days.	
Give oral Nifedipine 20 mg eight hourly for 48 hours. Total maximum dose of Nifedipine 60 mg/day.	
Monitor blood pressure and if the patient's blood pressure is less than 90/50, withhold Nifedipine dose and re-evaluate blood pressure in 15 minutes.	
If a patient experiences chest pain during Nifedipine therapy, discontinue Nifedipine, elevate the head of the bed, administer oxygen, and monitor FHR.	
There is insufficient evidence for any firm conclusion whether or not maintenance tocolytic therapy following threatened preterm labour is worthwhile. Thus maintenance therapy is not recommended.	
REPORTABLE CONDITIONS	
Consistent maternal hypotension (< 90/50) necessitating the withholding of Nifedipine, or if patient is symptomatic from the hypotension—dizziness, lightheaded, etc.	
Foetal bradycardia (< 120 bpm).	
Chest pain following Nifedipine administration.	
Uterine activity > 4 contractions/hour or as ordered by the physician.	

DOCUMENTATION	
All doses of Nifedipine should be recorded on the patient's drug chart.	
Document all side effects and/or adverse reactions to Nifedipine.	

Reference:

Tocolysis for women in preterm labour. National guideline. Available at; www.guideline.gov

Analgesia in Labour 40

FIRST STAGE	
Counselling in antenatal visits.	
Relaxation/breathing techniques during labour.	
Choice of narcotic analgesics	
Inj. Nalbuphine. 4 mg I/V SOS or 10 mg in 1 litre infusion in eight hours.	
Inj. Tramol. 30 mg I/V SOS or 100 mg in 1 litre infusion in eight hours.	
Inj. Stadol. 2 mg I/V in combination with Inj. Phenergan, it can be repeated after four hours interval.	
Antispasmodics	
Inj Spasfon/Inj Spasmex/Inj. Anafortan. (Phloroglucinol 40 mg, Trimethylphloroglucinol 04 mg) I/V or I/M, it can be given twice during first stage of labour.	
Inhalational methods	
Nitrous oxide. Entonox (50% nitrous oxide in oxygen) provides analgesia within 20–30 seconds of inhalation with a maximum effect after about 45 seconds.	
Epidural analgesia	
There are different techniques available for delivery of epidural analgesia.	
Single shot administration: A single dose of local anaesthetic injected through the epidural needle during labour may provide relatively fast onset of analgesia.	

Intermittent top-ups: Ideally a low dose mix of local anaesthetic and opioid is beneficial.	
SECOND STAGE	
Local infiltration. Local infiltration of perineum with lignocaine 1% before episiotomy.	

SECTION 03

STANDARD OPERATING PROCEDURES

Introduction to Standard Operating Procedures (SOPs)

Standard Operating Procedures are standardized written procedures, with detailed instructions. All SOPs for the department should be written in the same format with consistent font size, unit title, and section headers. It should include page numbers, date of initial approval, date it was effective within the department and date of revision if applicable. The body of the SOP at a minimum should include the objective of the SOP, definition of key terms and acronyms, defined list of responsible individuals and details outlining the procedures. It should also include the signature and date. Existing SOPs should be reviewed at regular intervals preferably annually to reassess and update. Distribution, education and training on new departmental SOPs should be consistent.

41 Coping with Hospital Admission High Risk Pregnancy

DESIRED PATIENT OUTCOMES	
Patients and their families in crisis will be supported appropriately.	
CLINICAL ASSESSMENT AND CARE	
Assess patient knowledge regarding reason for hospitalization and plan of care.	
Discuss with the patient, her perceptions of hospitalization, associated problems and possible solutions.	
Assess family reaction/adjustment to patient hospitalization.	
Identify those factors that might increase stress during the hospitalization (i.e. loss of income, child care, inadequate insurance, restructuring of roles).	
Provide a plan of care that allows patient's participation in management plan.	
Encourage the spouse and children to visit the patient.	
Provide interdisciplinary assistance when needed.	
Allow patient to express feelings openly and be non judgmental of coping mechanisms.	
PATIENT INSTRUCTIONS	
Instruct patient about the conditions and the consequences related to their antenatal diagnosis.	
Encourage patient to share any concerns, questions or fears she or her family is experiencing.	
Provide anticipatory guidance for delivery and/or discharge.	
DOCUMENTATION	
Document the relevant information.	
Document any complications during hospitalization.	

Four-Hour Obstetrical Hold—Short Stay Patients 42

INDICATIONS FOR SHORT STAY	
Blood pressure monitoring in patients with raised blood pressure.	
Decrease foetal movements.	
Confirmation of ruptured of membranes.	
Confirmation of labour in patients with previous history of preterm labour.	
OBSERVATIONS	
In patients with raised blood pressure: ○ B.P. monitoring hourly. ○ Sending relevant investigation.	
In patients with reduced foetal movements. ○ CTG. ○ AFI.	
Patient with suspicious of preterm labour. ○ Uterine contractions. ○ Foetal heart assessment.	
PROCEDURE	
Assess patient's understanding of need for evaluation and testing.	
Assess primary complaints of the patient.	
Obtain obstetrical history.	
Do general physical and abdominal examination.	
CTG must be reviewed and signed by obstetrician with date and time.	

Perform speculum and vaginal examination, if indicated.	
Obtain laboratory specimens if ordered.	
Clear discharge instructions and date of follow up visits.	
Counselling and provide information.	
Admit to inpatient status per protocol, if indicated.	
COUNSELLING AND INSTRUCTIONS	
Discuss the current status of patient.	
Satisfy the patient.	
Need for further monitoring.	
Give written follow up plan.	
DOCUMENTATION	
Complete four-hour hold record and document.	
Upon patient's four-hour hold discharge, send signed and labelled tracings with associated documentation to patient's record.	

43 Non-Stress Test

POLICY	
Non-stress test should be conducted for a minimum of 20 minutes.	
Patient should not be discharged until the CTG has been reviewed and signed by registrar and senior registrar in high risk pregnancy.	
CLINICAL ASSESSMENT AND CARE	
Take BP, pulse and temperature.	
Place the patient in dorsal position with a wedge on one side and attach the monitor.	
Instruct patient to press marker every time she perceives a foetal movement.	
A 20 minutes strip is sufficient for a reactive CTG.	
A 40 minutes strip is needed if CTG is not satisfactory.	
Biophysical Profile (BPP) is recommended in case of non-reactive CTG. Maintain FHR monitoring until BPP is initiated or tracing becomes reactive.	
Senior registrar must to be informed if CTG is non-reassuring.	
Regular uterine contractions during testing period should be mentioned.	
DOCUMENTATION	
Document CTG.	
CTG to be signed by registrar with name of the patient and date.	
A non reassuring CTG has to be signed by the senior registrar.	
In high risk patients CTG has to be signed by senior registrar.	

44 Epidural Analgesia During Labour

POLICY	
Epidural analgesia to be given by choice only not as compulsory during labour.	
DESIRED PATIENT OUTCOME	
The patient should be relieved of pain with minimal or no complications.	
CONTRAINDICATIONS	
Neurological abnormalities (i.e., multiple sclerosis) and history of back injuries.	
Abnormal coagulation profile.	
Skin infection at the site of insertion.	
Allergy to local anaesthesia.	
Sepsis, hypotension, bleeding.	
EFFECTS	
Sensory loss and motor loss.	
Hypotension.	
Shivering.	
Urinary retention.	
Nausea and vomiting (associated with hypotension).	
Dermatome sparing resulting in incomplete pain relief.	
COMPLICATIONS	
Post Dural Puncture Headache (PDPH).	
Nerve injury (extremely loss).	
Backache is a controversial issue as studies have shown labouring patients with or without epidural having the same incidence.	
Inflammation and haematoma at epidural site.	

EPIDURAL PLACEMENT AND ADMINISTRATION	
Things required	
Position adjustable bed.	
I/V stand.	
Pulse oximetry, Non invasive blood pressure monitoring.	
Epidural kit (16 G/18G).	
Epidural sterile drape set (Opsite, sterile gloves 6.5–8).	
Pyodine, Stenilium.	
Drugs: 2% xylocaine, 2% xylocaine with adrenaline, Bupivacaine.	
Emergency trolley: Atropine Adrenaline Ambo bag.	
Oxygen ports/cylinder.	
Oxygen masks.	
Methods of insertion	
Position: sitting or lying (right/left lateral).	
Monitoring.	
Identification of lumbar intervertebral space (usually L1–L5 preferably L2–3, L3–4).	
Paint and drape.	
Skin local anaesthetic infiltration.	
Epidural space identification by loss of resistance.	
Catheter insertion and positioning.	
Catheter fixation.	
Opsite dressing.	
Filter port attachment.	
Test dose: 2% xylocaine with adrenaline 3 ml (Heart rate monitoring).	
Injection of analgesic local anaesthetic dose.	
Local anaesthetic dosage	
Bolus of 0.1% Bupivacaine 10–20 ml (according to the pain score).	
Adjuvants e.g. Fentinyl can be added.	
Bupicaine epidural infusion can also be started.	

MONITORING

Monitoring of pulse

Initiate maternal pulse oximeter monitoring for initiation of epidural and each successive bolus dose.

Blood pressure

Check B.P. every five minutes during the epidural placement. After initiation of the block and with each successive dose, blood pressure must be taken at least every five minutes for 20 minutes and then every 15 minutes.

Position change

Position the patient either side—lying or sitting as planned by the anaesthesiologist.

Position patient initially flat, in a left lateral tilt with a hip wedge after epidural has been placed. Uterine displacement must be maintained throughout epidural anaesthesia to prevent hypotension and venacaval syndrome.

SPECIAL ISSUES

Blood pressure

During or after placement, if the patient's blood pressure falls by more than 30% of systolic pressure or 15% of diastolic pressure from baseline values prior to epidural placement:

- Secure left uterine displacement; preferably left lateral.
- Begin an IV bolus of 500 ml, preferably lactated ringers.
- Administer O2 at 10 L/min by face mask.
- Vasopressors e.g. Ephedrine 5 mg bolus may be given according to advice of anaesthesiologist.
- Notify anaesthetist immediately.
- Notify obstetric senior registrar.

Repeat BP at least every three minutes until stable.

Others

If the patient complains of inability to talk, peri-oral numbness, tinnitus, difficulty in breathing or appears confused or disoriented, frank convulsions may be imminent. Notify anaesthetist immediately and be prepared to ventilate patient with 100% oxygen and assist with manual ventilation.

Evaluate the catheter insertion site every eight hours for leakage or sign of inflammation.	
CARE OF EPIDURAL CATHETER	
Take extra care to prevent catheter displacement while shifting and positioning of patient.	
Only concerned anaesthetist is to give drugs by epidural catheter.	
Filter should always be attached.	
Avoid soiling of opsite dressing by blood, secretions etc.	
Instruction to the patient.	
○ Patient to stay in bed.	
○ Patient to have clear liquid diet.	
○ Inform concerned doctor in case of nausea, vomiting and motor loss.	
Epidural catheter can be retained in a patient for three days and also for LSCS and post op analgesia.	
REMOVAL OF EPIDURAL CATHETER	
Essentials	
Check site for haematoma, signs of inflammation and for sensory or motor loss.	
Blue top should be intact with the catheter.	
Documentation.	
Steps	
Peel off the adhesive dressing and ask the patient to lean forward, which will open the inter-vertebral space.	
Grasp the catheter with a gloved hand and attempt to withdraw the catheter smoothly. This should result in the catheter easily being withdrawn from the patient. If the catheter does not easily come out, do not persist attempting to remove it but rather consult the senior anaesthetist.	
After removal, examine the catheter tip and see a coloured mark at the end of the catheter.	
Clean the lumbar area with a clean cloth and apply dressing to the puncture site.	

Document the time of removal and the presence of tip of the catheter at the time of removal (proof of complete removal of epidural catheter).	
PATIENT EDUCATION	
Reinforce education about the purpose and use of epidural.	
Instruct the patient to report the following: ○ Unacceptable level of pain. ○ Pain at epidural site after removal. ○ Headache after epidural removal.	
FOLLOW UP	
Routine follow ups are not required, however follow-up with the anesthesiologist is advised in case of complaint.	
At the time of first post-natal visit, the attending doctor must examine the epidural site for signs of inflammation and infection.	
DOCUMENTATION	
Document the relevant information and complications.	
Document blue tip of epidural catheter on removal.	

Lithotomy Position 45

PRE-PROCEDURE	
Introduce, greet and explain the procedure.	
Explain the need for lithotomy position.	
Patients undergoing a procedure or during most vaginal deliveries will be placed in a lithotomy position.	
Assess if patient has areas of limited range of motion of joints before placing her in lithotomy position.	
Assess patient's skin integrity.	
PROCEDURE	
Assist patient, as needed, with lithotomy positioning just prior to vaginal delivery or procedure.	
Legs should be raised and lowered simultaneously to allow body to adjust to changes in circulatory blood volume and to prevent torsion injuries to the ligaments of the lower spine.	
Care should be taken to externally rotate the hip before abducting the leg.	
Legs and feet should be supported by the stirrup portion of the bed.	
The patient's buttocks should remain on the bed.	
Low lithotomy position is preferable.	
DOCUMENTATION	
Document the procedure.	

46 Perineal Scrub for Vaginal Delivery

POLICY	
Perform a perineal scrub before delivery.	
Exception will be made for precipitate delivery.	
EQUIPMENT	
Prep set should contain sponge holding forceps, Savlon swabs and gloves.	
PRE-PROCEDURE	
Explain the procedure to the patient.	
PROCEDURE	
Open disposable prep set using sterile technique.	
Wear gloves. Use first sponge to cleanse in the following manner: ○ Wipe across abdomen; turn sponge over. ○ Wipe leg beginning at inner aspect of thigh and continue outward. ○ Repeat for other leg. Discard sponge.	
Always use strokes that follow a direction away from the perineum.	
Use the second sponge to cleanse in the following manner: ○ Wipe either side of vaginal opening and center from top to bottom, turn sponge. ○ Cleanse the rectal area, discard sponge.	
POST-PROCEDURE	
Remove gloves.	
DOCUMENTATION	
Document the procedure.	

Care of the Newborn in the Delivery Room 47

POLICY	
The doctor should assess the neonate, at birth, preferably in the delivery room.	
Senior registrar neonatology should be called to attend all high-risk deliveries.	
DESIRED NEONATAL OUTCOMES	
Adequate respiration and thermoregulation should be established.	
CLINICAL ASSESSMENT AND CARE	
Dry infant thoroughly (heat loss can result in hypoxia).	
Suction of mouth and nose with a bulb sucker. Press bulb sucker before placing it in neonate's mouth.	
Give tactile stimulation and oxygen in cases of cyanosis.	
Clamp the umbilical cord an inch from skin surface and cut close to clamp, being careful to leave entire cord surface showing. Note the number of vessels in the cord and document.	
Document Apgar score at one and five minutes of age.	
Place identification tag on infant's wrist.	
Give injection Vitamin K intramuscularly.	
Initiate mother–neonate bonding by skin to skin contact between mother and neonate.	
REPORTABLE CONDITIONS	
Signs of immediate distress include:	
Respiratory distress, grunting, retracting or persistent respiratory rate of $>$ 60 breaths/minute.	
Heart rate $<$ 90 beats/minute, temperature $>$100° F.	
Generalized persistent central cyanosis.	
Abdominal distention.	

Convulsions.	
Two vessel cord.	
Congenital anomalies.	
DOCUMENTATION	
Document the time of delivery, Apgar score, vitamin K administered.	
Document the procedure.	

Care of the Patient with Neonatal Loss 48

DESIRED PATIENT OUTCOMES	
The patient and her family suffering a loss will be supported appropriately.	
CLINICAL ASSESSMENT AND CARE	
Assess patient's understanding and awareness of pregnancy loss.	
Assess for factors that may increase stress i.e. finances, care of siblings etc.	
Assess for symptoms of depression and psychosis and provide psychological support.	
Provide privacy for parents to see, hold the baby etc. if they so desire.	
Encourage open communication among family members and health care providers.	
Discuss how this loss might affect the family and relationships.	
Listen to the patient and respond appropriately.	
Do not create false hopes i.e. "you can have other children".	
Encourage patient to talk about her experience. Encourage verbalization of fears and feelings.	
Give factual information regarding the nature of the problem and the loss.	
Reassure the patient, allow her to cry and be patient with her anger.	
Offer multidisciplinary services, as psychiatry, genetic counselling and others.	
PATIENT INSTRUCTIONS	
Report depression.	
Provide written material when appropriate.	

Provide information on appropriate support groups.	
Decide about the next appointment.	
DOCUMENTATION	
Document the proceedings.	

49 Collection of Cord Blood Sample in Rh-Negative Mother

PROCEDURE	
After the delivery of the baby, 10 cc of cord blood sample is taken.	
Cord blood will be collected at delivery and labelled with the mother's name, date and time of collection.	
Hand over the sample to the attending doctor from the nursery for the following tests. o Blood group and Rh factor. o Serum bilirubin. o Haemoglobin. o Direct Coomb's test. o Reticulocyte count.	

50 Caesarean Section

POLICY	
Obstetric, neonatal and anaesthesia cover should be available to the labour and delivery unit 24 hours a day, seven days a week.	
For emergency caesarean section, the delivery should be performed as quickly and safely as possible best within 30 minutes of the decision to operate.	
In accordance with ACOG recommendations, the practice of elective caesarean delivery prior to 39 weeks gestation is not recommended.	
PREREQUISITES	
Documents vital signs.	
CTG tracing for 20 minutes.	
Informed consent must be signed before transferring to operation theatre.	
The surgical safety checklist must be utilized with every caesarean section.	
Disinfection and scrub protocol must be in place.	
Counselling of the patient regarding the caesarean delivery process and complications.	
Thromboprophylaxis, if indicated.	
DESIRED PATIENT OUTCOMES	
Safety of the patient and foetus will be maintained by aseptic measures.	
Delivery of the neonate should occur as quickly and safely as possible.	

CLINICAL ASSESSMENT AND CARE	
When the decision is made for an emergency caesarean delivery, all required personnel should be summoned stat to labour and delivery unit.	
Patients should be divided into high and low risk groups.	
High risk patients should be managed by senior registrar obstetrics, senior registrar anaesthesia and senior staff nurse and neonatologist and availability of ICU.	
Low risk patients should be managed by registrar obstetrics, registrar anaesthesia, staff nurse and neonatologist.	
Blood transfusion should be given only if needed.	
PATIENT INSTRUCTIONS	
Counselling.	
Investigations.	
Arrangement of blood.	
Informed consent.	
IMMEDIATE PRE–OP PREPARATION	
Prepare operating room before the arrival of the patient.	
Ensure proper functioning of equipment and presence of needed staff in operating theatre.	
Shift patient to operating theatre and transfer to operating table.	
Position of the patient as needed by anaesthesiologist.	
Place patient in supine position for surgery. ○ Place foam pillow under patient's head. ○ Place arms on arm boards, abducted at an angle less than or equal to 90°. ○ Place a wedge under right hip.	
DURING PROCEDURE	
Document the starting and ending time of the procedure.	
Sutures, instruments and linen are provided using aseptic technique.	

Monitor pulse, blood pressure, oxygen saturation during procedure.	
Obtain cord blood if Rh negative.	
Ensure proper cleansing of the patient and new-born identification.	
TRANSFER TO RECOVERY ROOM	
Before transferring to recovery room, ensure vital signs, spontaneous respiration, O_2 saturation, pain relief, urine and drain output.	
DOCUMENTATION	
Document exact time of delivery of infant and placenta.	
Complete operative record.	
Document the operation notes and post operative orders.	

51 Caesarean Section—Staff Nurse Responsibilities

PREREQUISITES	
Aseptic measures.	
Proper gowning and gloving technique.	
EQUIPMENT	
Instruments—Caesarean section set.	
Disposables.	
Sutures.	
Gloves.	
Light.	
Fluid warmer stand.	
PROCEDURE	
Open packs and instruments set.	
Add sutures, gloves and other equipment according to surgeon's preference.	
Scrub, gown and glove.	
Initiate and count as outlined in counts.	
Assist the procedure, being alert to follow sterile technique.	
Confirm final pack count.	
Nurse should be gowned and gloved, when removing drapes and soiled items.	
Use moist towels to clean skin around dressing site.	
Dressing will be placed on sterile field.	
Assist with transferring patient from table to stretcher.	

POST-PROCEDURE	
Room should be cleared of all soiled linens, drapes and instruments.	
Do not allow blood to dry on instruments.	
In the utility room, the instruments are soaked in chlorine solution and washed.	
DOCUMENTATION	
Document the proceedings.	

52 Use of Electro-Cautery During Operative Procedures

INTRODUCTION

Electro-cautery is the direct use of high-frequency electrical energy for controlled cutting, coagulation and desiccation of tissue. Mono-polar electro cautery requires a grounding pad, because the current must flow from the generator to the active electrode (pencil) through the patient to the grounding pad to return to the generator. Electrical burns are the greatest hazard of electro cautery. These burns are usually deeper than flame burns, causing widespread tissue necrosis and deep thrombosis.

DESIRED PATIENT OUTCOMES

The patient should not experience electrical burn/injury from electro-cautery unit.

GENERAL CARE

Assess for skin integrity of the area before pad placement.

Proper grounding pad application should include placement:

- On a long muscle mass as close to the incision as possible, i.e. upper lateral thigh. Away from the area to be operated, assuring the pad does not get wet.
- On an area free of hair, scars, or bony prominence.
- Of the entire pad in contact with the skin without gaps, folds or bends.

The electro-cautery pencil and patient ground wire are connected to the generator.

Set “Coag” and “Cut” settings.

Repeat assessment of skin integrity when pad is removed following the procedure.

REPORTABLE CONDITIONS	
Altered skin integrity—redness or broken areas, under the grounding pad.	
Malfunction of the unit.	
SAFETY MEASURES	
Ensure that the maintenance sticker is up-to-date.	
All equipment (generator, pencil, electrode, grounding pad) should be in working order.	
The grounding pad must be properly applied.	
Ensure that the patient is not in contact with any metal objects, i.e. stirrups or table.	
DOCUMENTATION	
Record the location of the grounding pad, the patient's skin condition before and after procedure, and the cutting and coagulation settings.	
Document any reportable condition.	

Prevention of Surgical Site Infection 53

PREREQUISITES	
Patient's privacy, appropriate light, couch and draw sheets (size: 1'x4' and 2'x 4').	
GENERAL INSTRUCTIONS	
Hair removal from surgical site, the night before surgery.	
Remove jewellery.	
Shower with an antiseptic soap, on the day of surgery. (home or hospital).	
Scrub the surgical area with Pyodine scrub for at least five minutes.	
Provide patient with gown.	
PREOPERATIVE INSTRUCTIONS	
Give preoperative IV antibiotics.	
Shift patient to preoperative room in operating theatre 30 minutes prior to surgery.	
Infected or colonized surgical personnel should not be allowed to operating theatre.	
SURGICAL TEAM INSTRUCTIONS	
Wearing a clean kit.	
Proper wash up technique has to be followed.	
Hair should be held back in a cap.	
Proper wash up and gowning technique should be followed.	

DURING SURGERY	
Avoid unnecessary tissue holding, moping and leaving bleeding points.	
POST OPERATIVE	
After completion of surgery, clean the operated area and surroundings of blood.	
Apply Pyodine to the sutured wound for five minutes, before application of dressing.	

Postoperative Care of the Patient After Gynaecological Surgery 54

DESIRED PATIENT OUTCOMES	
Patient should be free of complications during hospitalisation.	
Patient should report adequate pain control, using appropriate pain scale.	
CLINICAL ASSESSMENT AND CARE	
Assess pulse BP, temperature, respiration, pain, vaginal bleeding and surgical site at least every four hours for 24 hours, then every eight hours.	
Assess Foley catheter for patency and adequate urinary output four hourly.	
Encourage deep breathing.	
Assess IV site at least every four hours.	
Assess post-operative pain and pain management at least every 2–4 hours.	
Assess for bowel sounds at least every eight hours until flatus or bowel movement.	
Assess the ability to void spontaneously and adequately after Foley is discontinued. Assess until patient has two spontaneous voids $\geq$ 200 cc each.	
Assess incision site, at least every eight hours.	
Assist patient with her first out of bed experience.	
PATIENT INSTRUCTIONS	
Encourage patient to take oral fluids.	
Mobilization.	
DOCUMENTATION	
Document date and time of procedure.	
Document the complications, if any.	

55 Postoperative Pain Management in Major Gynaecological Procedures and Caesarean Section

Day 1	
One of the following medications can be used or multimodal pain management can be carried out	
Infusion Ringer's Lactate +2 ampoules of Lieometacin.	eight hourly
Inj. Nalbaine I/V infusion of 10 mg in 1 litre saline.	eight hourly
Inj. Paracetamol I/V 1 g.	eight hourly
Inj. Diclofenac I/M 75 mg.	12 hourly
Voltral suppository 100 mg.	12 hourly
Day 2	
Inj. Diclofenac 75 mg intramuscularly.	12 hourly
Voltral suppository 100 mg.	12 hourly
Day 3 to 7	
Tab. Diclofenac 50 mg.	eight hourly
Tab. Paracetamol 500 mg. (For patients with acid peptic disease)	eight hourly

PS: Multimodal pain management: More than one pain relieving agent has greater benefit in terms of pain relief rather than a single agent.

56 Instructions at Discharge—Normal Vaginal Delivery

GENERAL CARE
Drink plenty of water, at least eight glasses a day.
Take a high roughage diet and avoid constipation.
For constipation, Duphalac syrup, 30 ml at bedtime. The dose can be adjusted according to the requirement.
Sit as normally as possible. Sitting for the first time after delivery can be uncomfortable but eases after a couple of times.
Putting the baby to breast regularly helps establish normal breastfeeding.
Help should be sought for breastfeeding issues.
Bath can be taken a couple of hours after delivery.
The stitches take around ten days to heal and are self absorbing.
Sexual activity can be resumed after six weeks.
MEDICATION
Antibiotic has to be taken as instructed.
Cold pack can help alleviate pain of stitches.
Painkillers can be continued for additional days if pain is not settled.
Continue iron and calcium for at least three months after delivery.
PHYSICAL ACTIVITY AND EXERCISE
Regular physical activity can be resumed after 24 hours.
There is no restriction on climbing stairs.
Brisk walk and driving can be started once the soreness of the stitches settles down.
Abdominal and Kegel exercises should be started ten days after delivery and continued at least for three months.

FOLLOW-UP VISIT
It is important to visit for follow up to the clinic even if everything seems to be fine.
The visits are recommended at ten days and six weeks at the clinic.
Birth spacing of three years is recommended for most women.
Appropriate contraception should be planned for birth spacing and discussed with the doctor.
Risk factors in the pregnancy may need further management.
SPECIAL INSTRUCTIONS
In case of emergency, visit the labour room.
In case of minor issues, text on the cell number in the file.

Instructions at Discharge—Caesarean Section 57

GENERAL CARE
Drink plenty of water, at least eight glasses a day.
Take a high roughage normal diet and avoid constipation.
For constipation, Duphalac syrup, 30 ml at bedtime. The dose can be adjusted according to the requirement.
Walk as much as possible without getting exhausted. Stairs can be used regularly once the stitches are removed.
Putting the baby to breast regularly helps establish normal feeding.
Help should be sought for breastfeeding issues.
Bath can be taken a couple of days after caesarean section.
If the dressing becomes wet, it can be self changed.
Stitches will be removed on the eighth day in the labour room.
Sexual activity can be resumed after six weeks.
MEDICATION
Antibiotics have to be taken as instructed.
Cold pack can help alleviate pain of stitches.
Painkillers can be continued for additional days if pain is not settled.
Continue iron and calcium for at least three months after delivery.
PHYSICAL ACTIVITY AND EXERCISE
Regular physical activity can be resumed after seven days.
There is no restriction on climbing stairs and can be done regularly once the stitches are removed.
Kegel exercises should be started ten days after delivery and continued at least for three months.
Brisk walk and driving can be started six weeks after delivery.
Abdominal exercises should be resumed eight weeks.

FOLLOW-UP VISIT
It is important to visit for follow up to the clinic even if everything seems to be fine.
The visits are recommended at three and six weeks at the clinic.
Birth spacing of three years is recommended for most women.
Appropriate contraception should be planned for birth spacing and discussed with the doctor.
Risk factors in the pregnancy may need further management.
SPECIAL INSTRUCTIONS
In case of minor issues, text on the cell number in the file.
Thromboprophylaxis if initiated should be continued six weeks after surgery.
In case of emergency, visit the hospital.
Report in case of the following issues. ○ Fever more than 100.5° F. ○ Problems with the wound. ○ Heavy bleeding. ○ Severe nausea or pain. ○ Any unusual symptoms.

58 Instructions at Discharge—Major Gynaecological Procedure

GENERAL CARE
Drink plenty of water, at least eight glasses a day.
Take a high roughage normal diet and avoid constipation.
For constipation, Duphalac syrup, 30 ml at bedtime. The dose can be adjusted according to the requirement.
Walk as much as possible without getting exhausted. Stairs can be used regularly once the stitches are removed.
Bath can be taken a couple of days after surgery.
If the dressing becomes wet, it can be self changed.
Keep the incision clean and dry.
Stitches will be removed on the eighth day.
Sexual activity can be resumed after six weeks.
MEDICATION
Antibiotics have to be taken as instructed.
Cold pack can help alleviate pain of stitches.
Painkillers can be continued for additional days if pain is not settled.
Take the vitamins and supplements as instructed.
PHYSICAL ACTIVITY AND EXERCISE
Regular physical activity can be resumed after seven days.
There is no restriction on climbing stairs and can be done regularly once the stitches are removed.
Brisk walk and driving can be started in six weeks.
Abdominal exercises should be resumed eight weeks.
FOLLOW-UP VISIT
It is important to come for follow up even if everything seems to be fine.

Histopathology report should be presented at the first follow up visit.
The follow up visits are recommended at three and six weeks.
Referral to physician in case of medical disorder.
SPECIAL INSTRUCTIONS
Thromboprophylaxis if initiated should be continued six weeks after surgery.
In case of emergency, visit the hospital.
Report in case of the following issues. ○ Fever more than 100.5° F. ○ Problems with the wound. ○ Heavy bleeding. ○ Severe nausea or pain. ○ Any unusual symptoms.

59 Instructions at Discharge—Minor Gynaecological Procedure

GENERAL CARE
Drink plenty of water, at least eight glasses a day.
Take a high roughage normal diet and avoid constipation.
There is no restriction to mobility.
Sexual activity can be resumed depending on the minor procedure performed.
MEDICATION
Antibiotics have to be taken as instructed.
Cold pack can help alleviate pain of stitches. (If need be).
Painkillers can be continued for additional days if pain is not settled.
PHYSICAL ACTIVITY AND EXERCISE
Regular physical activity can be resumed after mobilisation.
There is no restriction on climbing stairs.
Brisk walk and driving can be resumed after 48 hours.
FOLLOW-UP VISIT
It is important to come for follow up even if everything seems to be fine.
Follow up visit is recommended at two weeks.
Histopathology report should be presented at the follow up visit.
SPECIAL INSTRUCTIONS
In case of ERPC, appropriate contraception has to be discussed and decided.

60 Instructions at Discharge—Diagnostic Laparoscopy

GENERAL CARE
Drink plenty of water, at least eight glasses a day.
Take a high roughage normal diet and avoid constipation.
There is no restriction to mobility.
The patient should be informed that she can experience shoulder tip pain.
Stitch can be removed on the eighth day if required.
Sexual activity can be resumed after ten days.
MEDICATION
Antibiotic has to be taken as instructed.
Cold pack can help alleviate pain of stitches.
Painkillers can be continued for additional days if pain is not settled.
PHYSICAL ACTIVITY AND EXERCISE
Regular physical activity can be resumed after two days.
There is no restriction on climbing stairs.
Brisk walk and driving can be started after two days.
Abdominal exercises should be resumed four weeks.
FOLLOW-UP VISIT
It is important to come for follow up even if everything seems to be fine.
The follow up visits are recommended at two and six weeks.
Next steps and further plan of management should be decided at the follow up visit with mutual consultation.
SPECIAL INSTRUCTIONS
In case of emergency, visit the hospital.

Infection Prevention—Components 61

Practices and procedures that limit the transmission of infectious agents to patients, staff and the community.
COMPONENTS OF INFECTION PREVENTION
Use of personal protective equipment.
Hand washing.
Gloving.
Proper aseptic technique during procedures.
Use of antiseptics.
Sterilization and disinfection.
Housekeeping and waste disposal.
USE OF PERSONAL PROTECTIVE EQUIPMENT
Use of cap, mask, gloves, gowns, high boots and protective glasses.
HAND WASHING
Hand washing with plain soap or antiseptic soap and running water for patient examination.
Use of alcohol base hand rubs, before and after patient examination.
SCRUBBING
Hand scrubbing (for five minutes before procedures with pyodine or sterilium). ○ Rub hand palm to palm. ○ Right palm over left dorsum with interlaced fingers and vice versa. ○ Palm to palm with fingers interlaced. ○ Backs of fingers to opposing palms with fingers interlocked. ○ Rotational rubbing of left thumb clasped in tight palm and vice versa. ○ Rotational rubbing, backwards and forwards with clasped fingers of right hand in left palm and vice versa.

GLOVING
Wear gloves (clean, non-sterile) when touching blood, body fluids, secretions, excretions or mucous membranes.
Change gloves between contacts with different patients.
Change gloves between tasks/procedures on the same patient to prevent cross contamination between different body sites.
Remove gloves immediately after use and before attending to another patient.
Use sterilized surgical gloves for all operative procedures.
Sterile surgical gloves can become contaminated and needs change: ○ If the outside of a sterile glove is touched with an ungloved hand. ○ If face or clothing outside the sterile field is touched. ○ If the glove becomes torn or punctured.
ASEPTIC TECHNIQUE DURING PROCEDURES
Avoid unnecessary tissue handling, moping and leaving bleeding points.

62 Infection Prevention—Steps

GENERAL INSTRUCTIONS FOR PATIENTS
Hair removal **from surgical site,** a night before surgery.
Remove jewelry.
Shower with an antiseptic soap on the day of surgery. (home or hospital).
Scrub the surgical area with Pyodine scrub for at least five minutes.
Provide patient with gown.
PREOPERATIVE INSTRUCTION
Give preoperative IV antibiotics acceding to the hospital protocol and need of the patient.
Infected or colonized surgical personnel should not be allowed to operating theatre.
DURING SURGERY
Avoid unnecessary tissue holding, moping and leaving bleeding points.
POSTOPERATIVE
After completion of surgery, clean the operated area and surroundings of blood.
Apply Pyodine to the sutured wound for five minutes, before application of dressing.

63 Infection Prevention—Disinfection and Sterilization

DISINFECTION

A disinfection process is one that intended to significantly reduce the number of pathogenic microorganisms on instruments by removing and/or killing them.
MATERIAL REQUIRED
Kidney tray with instruments, pair of gloves and small towel.
A plastic bucket with clean water.
A plastic bucket with 0.5% chlorine solution.
Sterilizer.
PREPARATION OF 0.5% CHLORINE SOLUTION
One part of bleach and nine parts of water.
STEPS FOR INSTRUMENT PROCESSING
Step 1 (Decontamination). ○ Soak in 0.5% chlorine solution for 10 minutes before cleansing. ○ Rinse or wash immediately.
Step 2 (Cleaning). ○ Using a brush, wash with soap and water. ○ Rinse with clean water. ○ Air or towel dry.
Step 3 (HLD). ○ Steam or boil for 20 minutes. ○ Chemically HLD by soaking in 0.5% chlorine solution for 20 minutes. ○ Rinse well with boiled water and air dry before use.

STERILIZATION

Sterilization process is one that eliminates microbiological organisms to achieve a sepsis. After the step one and step two of the disinfection, follow the methods for sterilization:	
Steam	(For heat stable instruments 100°c for 20 minutes).
Dry heat	(For heat stable instruments 180°c for 30 min).
Chemical	(For heat labile instruments 0.5% chlorine for 20 min).
OPERATION THEATER DISINFECTION PROTOCOL	
Carbolize the operation theatre walls daily.	
Turn on ultraviolet light in the operating theatre for 6–8 hours daily, at night.	
Fumigation should be done once a month.	
Swabs should be taken from operating theatre area every three months for culture and sensitivity of microorganisms.	
Operating theatre equipment is cleaned with 2.5% alkaline Glutraldehyde solution, every day.	
Instruments should be dipped for 10 minutes in 2.5% alkaline Glutraldehyde solution 10 g/l daily.	
Instruments should be autoclaved at least for 20–30 minutes, before every use.	
HOUSE KEEPING AND WASTE DISPOSAL	
Clean up after any procedure.	
Dispose of waste in a leak proof container.	
Wipe surfaces using cloth and 0.5% chlorine solution.	
Dispose of sharps in puncture proof container.	
FOUR COMPONENTS OF WASTE MANAGEMENT	
Sorting. Separating waste by type at the place where it is generated.	

Handling. Collecting and transporting waste within the facility.
Interim storage. Storing waste within the facility until it can be disposed of.
Final disposal. Eliminating or transporting solid medical waste, liquid medical waste, sharps, and hazardous chemical waste from the health facility.

SECTION 04

PATIENT SAFETY CHECKLIST

Introduction to Patient Safety Checklist

Patient safety is a new healthcare discipline that emphasizes the reporting, analysis, and prevention of medical errors that often leads to adverse health care events

Patient safety goals

The purpose of the patient safety goals is to improve patient safety. The goals focus on problems in health care safety and how to solve them.

1. **Identify patients correctly**
   a. Use at least two ways to identify patients. For example, use the patient's name and date of birth. This is done to make sure that each patient gets the correct medicine and treatment.
   b. Make sure that the correct patient gets the correct blood when they get a blood transfusion.
2. **Improve staff communication**
   Get important test results to the right staff person on time.
3. **Use medicines safely**
   a. Before a procedure, label medicines that are not labeled. For example, medicines in syringes.
   b. Take extra care of patients on anticoagulants
   c. Record and pass along correct information about a patient's medicines. Find out what medicines the patient is taking. Compare those medicines to new medicines given to the patient. Make sure the patient knows which medicines to take when they are at home.
4. **Use alarms safely**
   Make improvements to ensure that alarms on medical equipment are heard and responded to on time.
5. **Prevent infection**
   a. Use the hand cleaning guidelines from the World Health Organization. Set and use goals for improving hand cleaning.

b. Use proven guidelines to prevent infections, which are difficult to treat, from IV or central lines, from surgery and from urinary catheterization.

6. **Identify patient safety risks**

   Find out which patients are most likely to try to commit suicide.

7. **Prevent mistakes in surgery**

   a. Make sure that the correct surgery is done on the correct patient and at the correct place on the patient's body.

   b. Mark the correct place on the patient's body where the surgery is to be done.

   c. Pause before the surgery to make sure that a mistake is not being made.

Patient safety indicators

The Agency for Healthcare Research and Quality issued a list of 20 "Patient Safety Indicators (PSI's)". The following list consists of these indicators, all of which highlight the most common areas for hospital and medical errors to occur.

1. **Complications of anaesthesia**

   a. Reaction to anaesthetic agent used during surgery.

   b. Complications from airways may cause problems such as coughing, gagging or muscle spasms in the larynx

   c. Insertion of airway may cause hypertension and tachycardia

   d. Other complications may include damage to teeth and lips, swelling in the larynx, sore throat and hoarseness caused by injury or irritation of the larynx.

2. **Death in low-mortality cases**

   This indicator is intended to identify in-hospital deaths in patients unlikely to die during hospitalization.

3. **Decubitus ulcer**

   This results from pressure on the skin, typically in patients during hospital recovery or whose mobility is limited in bed.

4. **Failure to rescue**

   When a patient dies following the development of a complication. The underlying assumption is that good hospitals identify these complications quickly and treat them aggressively.

5. **Foreign body left during procedure**

   These may occur when a foreign body is accidentally left in a patient during a procedure. For example, instruments. The patient may or may not feel any symptoms.

6. **Iatrogenic pneumothorax**

   Caused by accidentally puncture the lung during a surgical procedure. Symptoms include chest pain,dysnoea, bradycardia and numbness in hands and fingers.

7. **Infections due to medical care, provider level**

   a. Cases of infection due to medical care, primarily those related to Intravenous (IV) lines and catheters. Patients with potential immunocompromised states are excluded.

   b. This indicator includes children and neonates. It should be noted that high-risk neonates are at particularly high risk for catheter-related infections.

8. **Postoperative hip fracture**

   These cases involve in-hospital fractures, specifically hip fractures. It excludes patients in MDC 8 (musculoskeletal disorders) and patients with indications for trauma or cancer, or principal diagnoses of seizure, syncope, stroke, coma, cardiac arrest or poisoning, as these patients may have a fracture present on admission.

9. **Postoperative haemorrhage or haematoma**

   This indicator is intended to capture cases of haemorrhage or haematoma following a surgical procedure when it is unexpected.

10. **Postoperative physiologic and metabolic derangement**

    Cases of postoperative metabolic or physiologic complications after elective surgery.

11. **Postoperative respiratory failure**

    Respiratory failure can occur after any surgical procedure. Symptoms include coughing, tightness in the chest and wheezing.

12. **Postoperative pulmonary embolism or deep vein thrombosis**

    A blood clot that occurs in the lung after any surgical procedure. A pulmonary embolism is a blood clot that forms in another part of the body and then travels to the lung and causes a blockage. A pulmonary embolism can cause permanent lung damage due to lack of blood flow and insufficient oxygen supply. A deep vein thrombosis is a blood clot that occurs in deeper veins in the thigh or calf that can be very painful.

13. **Postoperative sepsis:**

    Sepsis may be associated with clinical symptoms of illness, such as fever, chills, malaise, low blood pressure and mental status changes. Sepsis can be a serious situation, a life threatening disease calling for urgent and comprehensive care

14. **Postoperative wound healing**

    The wound breaks down and healing can be very lengthy and difficult and the risk of infection is high. Risk factors for the condition include diabetes, increased age, obesity, wound infection, poor wound closing and injury to the wound following the operation. Symptoms include abdominal pain, vomiting, diarrhea and wound discharge.

15. **Accidental puncture or laceration**

    When an unexpected puncture or laceration occurs during surgery. If it is not corrected it could be life threatening due to loss of blood and decreased function from lacerated part.

16. **Transfusion reaction**

    When a person has an allergic reaction to the transfusion of blood products.Symptoms include anxiety, chest and/or back pain, jaundice, fever and chills.

17. **Birth trauma—injury to neonate**

    Birth trauma for infants born alive in a hospital. This excludes patients born pre-term, as birth trauma in these patients may be less preventable than for full-term infants. Some examples of trauma for infants are jaundice, asphyxia, brain damage and infection.

18. **Obstetric trauma—vaginal delivery with instrument**

    Potentially preventable trauma during vaginal delivery with instrument. Some examples of trauma for infants are jaundice, asphyxia, brain damage and infection.

19. **Obstetric trauma—vaginal delivery without Instrument**

    Potentially preventable trauma during a vaginal delivery. Some examples of trauma for infants are jaundice, asphyxia, brain damage and infection.

20. **Obstetric trauma—cesarean delivery**

    Potentially preventable trauma during Cesarean delivery. Some examples of trauma for infants are jaundice, asphyxia, brain damage and infection.

References

1. Patient Safety Indicators (PSIs)—Institute for Healthcare Improvement. At www.ihi.org/resources/Pages/.../PatientSafetyIndicatorsPSIs.aspx
2. 2015 National Patient Safety Goals; at www.jointcommission.org/standards_information/npsgs.aspx

64 Induction of Labour (IOL)

Patient Safety Checklist

BASIC INFORMATION	
Gravida and parity.	
Expected date of delivery.	
Duration of pregnancy.	
INDICATION FOR INDUCTION	
Indication should be known.	
Decision at senior registrar level.	
RISK FACTORS	
Medical conditions and issues with foetoplacental units such as Intra Uterine Growth Restriction (IUGR), decrease liquor, decrease foetal heart rate.	
Known allergies.	
Risk factors for anaesthesia.	
Pertinent laboratory tests.	
PREREQUISITES	
Cephalic presentation.	
Pelvic assessment and Bishop score.	
Definitive indication.	
Pregnancy preferably 39 weeks.	
In cases of duration of gestation less than 39 weeks, decision by senior registrar.	
Use of Dexamethasone if induction prior to 39 weeks.	
Counselling about need, method and possible outcome.	
Consent from patient.	

SELECTION OF METHOD	
Prostaglandin gel.	
Misoprostol.	
Oxytocin.	

Bishop scoring system

Score	Dilation (cm)	Position of Cervix	Effacement (%)	Station*	Cervical Consistency
0	Closed	Posterior	0–30	-3	Firm
1	1–2	Midposition	40–50	-2	Medium
2	3–4	Anterior	60–70	-1, 0	Soft
3	5–6		80	+1, +2	-

*Station reflects a -3 to+3 scale.

References

Induction of labour. ACOG Practice Bulletin No. 107. American College of Obstetricians and Gynaecologists. Obstet Gynaecol 2009; 114:386–97.

65 Trial of Labour After Previous Caesarean Delivery (TOLAC)

Patient Safety Checklist

BASIC INFORMATION	
Gravida and parity.	
LMP and EDD.	
Duration of pregnancy—confirmed.	
INTEGRITY OF SCAR	
Previous caesarean section—indication, complications, stage of labour, outcome, postoperative infection, foetal weight.	
Documentation of previous caesarean section.	
Type of uterine incision.	
Current pregnancy—risk factors, estimated foetal weight and amount of liquor.	
COUNSELLING	
Patient is provided with information about TOLAC.	
Counselling about the risks, benefits, chances of success, and alternatives of TOLAC.	
The patient is informed of the time that the facility on an average takes for availability of operation theatre to perform an emergency Caesarean Section.	
Chances of success of VBAC.	
INFORMED CONSENT	
After discussing the pros and cons the patient and her health care provider have concluded that the patient continues to be an appropriate candidate for TOLAC.	
Patient has signed a consent form for TOLAC and emergency Caesarean delivery.	

HEALTH CARE TEAM	
A nurse midwife, OB/G doctor, anaesthesiologist, paediatrician and appropriate nursing staff.	
ABSOLUTE CONTRAINDICATION	
Use of Misoprostol.	

References

1. Vaginal birth after previous Caesarean delivery. Committee Opinion No. 115. American College of Obstetricians and Gynaecologists. Obstet Gynaecol 2010;116:450–63.

66 Planned Caesarean Section

Patient Safety Checklist

PREREQUISITES	
Gravida, parity and complications in previous pregnancy and delivery.	
Confirm duration of pregnancy and indication.	
Betamethasone or Dexamethasone if caesarean section is performed before 39 weeks.	
Risk factors as anaemia, hypertension, diabetes.	
In case of risk for excessive bleeding, adequate blood and blood products arranged, blood bank and hospital administration informed.	
Blood group of the patient must be known.	
Document allergies, drug reactions and prior blood transfusion reactions.	
Relevant investigations including CBC and screening for hepatitis B, hepatitis C and HIV.	
Counselling and informed consent.	
Anaesthetic preoperative assessment and consent.	
Anaesthetic plan.	
Steps to reduce surgical and anaesthetic risk.	
Surgical site disinfection plan.	
DAY OF SURGERY	
Bath and use of Pyodine scrub on surgical site for at least five minutes.	
DVT prophylaxis if needed.	
Inform paediatrics. For high risk patients, senior registrar to receive baby.	
Document foetal heart rate.	

Before the start of surgery, name of patient, indication and consent and blood group of patient must be confirmed.	
Before start of surgery, risk factors and role of team members needs reconfirmation.	
Team follow proper wash up technique.	
Paint surgical site and surrounding area with Pyodine and let it dry at least for three minutes.	
Antibiotic prophylaxis at the time of incision.	
DURING SURGERY	
Pack and instrument counts performed before incision and are reconfirmed before closing the abdomen.	
POSTOPERATIVE	
Document visual assessment of blood loss.	
Document operative findings, notes and complications.	
Document baby notes including A/S.	
Confirm patient is awake.	
Adequate pain relief.	
Review and document satisfactory patient condition before shifting.	

References

1. Patient safety in the surgical environment. Committee Opinion No. 464. American College of Obstetricians and Gynaecologists. Obstet Gynaecol 2010;116:786–90
2. Antimicrobial prophylaxis for Caesarean delivery: Timing of administration. Committee Opinion No. 465. American College of Obstetricians and Gynaecologists. Obstet Gynaecol 2010;116:791–2.
3. Foetal lung maturity. ACOG Practice Bulletin No. 97. American College of Obstetricians and Gynaecologists. Obstet Gynaecol 2008;112:717–26

67 Pregnancy Risk Assessment

A pregnancy at risk of serious complications is considered to be a high risk pregnancy. This pregnancy may be identified by using a scoring system such as developed by Hobel et al. The risk factors are assigned a score corresponding to a degree of risk. A total score of 10 or more indicates a high risk pregnancy that should receive more than routine prenatal care.

OBSTETRIC HISTORY RISK FACTOR	Points
Previous stillbirth	10
Previous neonatal death	10
Previous premature infant	10
Post-term > 42 weeks	10
Foetal blood transfusion for haemolytic disease	10
Repeated miscarriages	5
Previous infant > 10 pounds	5
Six or more completed pregnancies	5
History of eclampsia	5
Previous Caesarean section	5
History of preeclampsia	1
History of foetus with anomalies	1
MEDICAL HISTORY RISK FACTOR	**Points**
Abnormal PAP test	10
Chronic hypertension	10
Heart disease NYHA Class II-IV (symptomatic)	10
Insulin dependent diabetes (≥ A2)	10
Moderate to severe renal disease	10
Previous endocrine ablation	10
Sickle cell disease	10

Epilepsy	5
Heart disease NYHA Class I (no symptoms)	5
History of TB or PPD >= 10 mm	5
Positive serology (for syphilis)	5
Pulmonary disease	5
Thyroid disease	5
FAMILY HISTORY RISK FACTOR	**Points**
Family history of diabetes	1

PHYSICAL RISK FACTOR	Points
Incompetent cervix	10
Uterine malformations	10
Maternal age 35 and over or 15 and under	5
Maternal weight <100 pounds or >200 pounds	5
Small pelvis	5
CURRENT PREGNANCY RISK FACTOR	**Points**
Abnormal foetal position	10
Moderate to severe preeclampsia	10
Multiple pregnancy	10
Placenta abruption	10
Placenta previa	10
Polyhydramnios or oligohydramnios	10
Excessive use of drugs/alcohol	5
Gestational diabetes (A1)	5
Kidney infection	5
Mild preeclampsia	5
Rh sensitization only	5
Severe anaemia < 9 g/dL hemoglobin	5
Severe flu syndrome or viral disease	5
Vaginal spotting	5

Bladder infection	1
Emotional problems	1
Mild anaemia 9 g/dL hemoglobin	1
Moderate alcohol use	1
Smoking >= one pack per day	1

Reference:

Hobel CJ, Hyvarinen MA et al. Prenatal and intrapartum high-risk screening. Am J Obstet Gynaecol. 1973; 117: 1–9. PMID: 4722373

SECTION 05

GUIDELINES AND PROTOCOLS

Introduction to Guidelines and Protocols

Guidelines and protocols consist of two distinct components: the evidence summary and the detailed instructions for the application of that evidence to patient care [8]. For the common healthcare provider, clinical practice guidelines are systematically developed statements that assist decisions about appropriate health care for specific circumstances. They are rigorously developed using evidence-based medicine criteria. The guidelines have been locally adapted to suit our local circumstances and to achieve a feeling of ownership, both of which are important factors in guideline uptake and use.

At the end of each guideline, protocol of that topic is also given, for easy reading, quick reference and easy implementation.

68 Guideline Management of HIV in Pregnancy

Adapted from Green Top Guideline No. 30 June 2010

1. PURPOSE

The purpose of this guideline is to reduce mother to child transmission and improve strategies of maternal screening and maternal health with HIV in pregnancy.

2. BACKGROUND

HIV is a retrovirus containing reverse transcriptase. HIV targets lymphocytes expressing CD4 lymphocytes, causing immunosuppression. When CD4 lymphocytes fall below a critical level, infected individuals become more susceptible to opportunistic infections and malignancies.

Routes of transmission of HIV
Sexual intercourse
Blood transfusion
Blood products
Injections
From mother to child
Breastfeeding

Treatment is with a combination of three or more anti-retroviral drugs, known as Highly Active Anti-Retroviral Therapy (HAART)

2.1. Risks of mother-to-child transmission in untreated women

The risk of mother-to-child transmission of HIV is between 15% and 20% in non-breastfeeding women and between 25% and 40% in breastfeeding woman.

The obstetric factors associated with transmission
Mode of delivery
Duration of membrane rupture
Delivery before 32 weeks

In the absence of breastfeeding, 80% of transmissions occur perinatally, around the time of labour and delivery.

Breastfeeding doubles the risk of mother-to-child transmission from around 14% to 28%.

2.2. Risk of mother-to-child transmission in treated women

Transmission rate of less than 2% is observed by

- HAART.
- Elective caesarean section.
- Avoidance of breastfeeding.

3. ANTENATAL HIV SCREENING

3.1. What can be done to ensure continued high uptake of HIV screening?

All pregnant women are recommended to have screening for HIV infection in every pregnancy at their booking antenatal visit.	A
All pregnant women who are HIV positive should be managed by a multidisciplinary team.	D
If a woman declines screening, her reasons should be explored, the decision to decline screening should be documented and screening offered again at around 28 weeks.	✓
All women booking for antenatal care should be tested for HIV, syphilis, rubella and hepatitis.	B

3.2. What type of HIV test should be used?

Fourth-generation laboratory assays are recommended as the first-line HIV test for antenatal screening.	D

Fourth generation tests include testing for HIV antibody and p24 antigen.

A reactive result on initial testing is always confirmed by testing the same sample with two further assays.

When the patient has her HIV screening test at 26 weeks of gestation or later, an urgent requestshould be made and the result issued by the laboratory within 24 hours. D

Rapid HIV tests are done for women with unknown HIV status who present in labour. D

3.3. How can seroconversions in pregnancy be prevented and identified?

All women testing HIV negative at booking should be informed about safe sex and high risks scenarios for HIV transmission.

Repeat testing should be available at any time during pregnancy.

Women at continued high risk of HIV acquisition should be offered a repeat HIV test. D

3.4. How should HIV test results be recorded and communicated?

Doctors reviewing women during antenatal care should ensure that the HIV result is clearly documented. D

4. PROFESSIONAL APPROACH TO THE ANTENATAL CARE OF WOMEN WHO ARE HIV POSITIVE

4.1. What is the role of the multidisciplinary team and who should it include?

All antenatal care for women who are HIV positive should be managed by a multidisciplinary team, including an HIV physician, obstetrician, specialist midwife, health advisor and paediatrician. D

4.2. What are the psychosocial and ethical issues?

Pregnant women should be reassured that their confidentiality will be maintained. D

Care must be taken to avoid disclosure to a woman's partner or family members. ✓

Women who are HIV positive should be advised about safer-sex practices and the use of condoms, to prevent transmission of HIV and other sexually transmitted infections to an uninfected partner. B

Consistent use of condoms is associated with an 80% reduction in transmission of HIV.

Women should be encouraged to disclose their HIV status to their partner and should be given appropriate support. Women with existing children of unknown HIV status should be tested for HIV. D

5. INTERVENTIONS TO PREVENT DISEASE PROGRESSION IN THE MOTHER AND PREVENT MOTHER-TO-CHILD TRANSMISSION OF HIV

5.1. What interventions prevent disease progression in the mother?

Women who require HIV treatment for their own health should take HAART and should continue treatment following delivery. A

The timing of initiation of HAART is important:

Delaying treatment until the CD4 lymphocyte count has fallen below 200×106/l is associated witha greater risk of disease progression and death.

Indications of HAART:

Symptomatic HIV infection.

CD4 count less than 350 x 10^6/L.

CD4 count less than 200 x 10^6/L HAART+prophylaxis against.

PCP (Pneumocystis Pneumonia).

5.2. What interventions prevent mother-to-child transmission of HIV?

5.2.1. Avoidance of breastfeeding

All women who are HIV positive should be advised to avoid breastfeeding. B

5.2.2. Antiretroviral therapy

All pregnant HIV positive women should be advised to take antiretroviral therapy:

a. For women who require HIV treatment for their own health, should continue HAART throughout pregnancy and postpartum. A

b. For women who do not require HIV treatment for their own health, HAART should be initiated between 20 and 28 weeks and discontinued at delivery. B

c. For women who do not require HIV treatment for their own health, with viral load less than 10,000 copies/ml and are to be delivered by elective caesarean section, an alternative to HAART is Zidovudine monotherapy given between 20 and 28 weeks, given orally twice daily, intravenously at delivery and discontinued immediately thereafter. A

Zidovudine (ZDV) monotherapy (ZDV given as a single agent) is the only anti-retroviral agent thathas been shown to reduce significantly the risk of mother-to-child transmission in a randomized controlled trial.

5.2.3. Mode of delivery

Delivery by elective caesarean section at 38 weeks to prevent labour and/or ruptured membranes is recommended for:

Women taking HAART and plasma viral load greater than 50 copies/ml	A
Women taking ZDV monotherapy as an alternative to HAART	A
Women with HIV and hepatitis C co-infection	D

Delivery by elective caesarean section for obstetric indications or maternal request should be delayed uptil 39 completed weeks of gestation in women with plasma viral loads of less than 50 copies/ml, to reduce the risk of transient tachypnoea of the newborn. D

A planned vaginal delivery can be offered to women taking HAART with plasma viral loads of less than 50 copies/ml. B

6. ANTENATAL CARE FOR PREGNANT WOMEN WHO ARE HIV POSITIVE

6.1. What antenatal blood tests for infections are recommended for women who are HIV positive?

Women who are HIV positive are recommended to have a screening blood test for syphilis, hepatitis B and rubella in every pregnancy at their booking antenatal visit. D

Additional blood tests for women who are HIV positive include hepatitis C, varicella zoster, measles and toxoplasma. D

Women who are HIV positive taking HAART at the time of booking should be screened for gestational diabetes. D

6.2. What immunizations should be undertaken?

Hepatitis B, pneumococcal and influenza immunization are recommended for all who are HIV positive; these immunizations can be safely administered in pregnancy. D

6.3. When should screening for genital infections be undertaken?

Women who are HIV positive should be screened for genital infections at booking and again at 28 weeks. Any infection detected should be treated even if asymptomatic. D

6.4. How should screening for aneuploidy be undertaken?

Screening for aneuploidy should be done in a routine manner. D

6.5. How safe is invasive diagnostic testing?

Women who are HIV positive considering invasive diagnostic testing should be counseled in a foetal medicine unit and with HIV physician regarding the risk of HIV transmission. D

6.6. When should ultrasound scanning be undertaken?

Dating and anomaly scans should be done. D

6.7. What additional monitoring is necessary?

Plasma viral load.
Drug toxicities.
CBC.
Urea.
Electrolytes.
Liver function test.

6.8. When should a decision regarding mode of delivery be taken?

A plan regarding mode of delivery should be made at 36 weeks following detailed discussion with the mother. D

Women taking HAART who have a viral load of less than 50 copies/ml at 36 weeks may be offered a planned vaginal delivery.

For women taking HAART with a viral load of less than 50 copies/ml who want caesarean section should be done at 39+weeks, to minimize the risk of transient tachypnoea of the newborn.

For women with a viral load greater than 50 copies/ml and those taking ZDV monotherapy as an alternative to HAART, caesarean section should be done at 38 weeks; in these women, earlier delivery is done because the risk of perinatal HIV transmission associated with labour and/or ruptured membranes is more serious than the risk of transient tachypnoea.

7. MANAGEMENT OF ANTENATAL COMPLICATIONS

7.1. What are the complications of HIV and adverse effects of HAART?

Side effects of HAART
Gastrointestinal. disturbances.
Skin rashes.
Hepatotoxicity.
Lactic acidosis.

B

HIV-related complications should also be considered as a cause of acute illness in pregnant women whose HIV status is unknown. In these circumstances, rapid HIV testing should be done. D

Presentation with symptoms suggestive of pre-eclampsia, cholestasis or other signs of liver dysfunction may indicate drug toxicity

7.2. What is the risk of preterm delivery?

Women should be counseled about the increased risk of preterm delivery associated with HAART.

7.3. How should preterm labour be managed?

For women presenting with threatened preterm labour, initial assessment should be done in a routine manner. The multidisciplinary team should be involved so that a clear plan of care is made. D

a. The usual indications for steroids apply.

b. A genital infection screen should be done.

c. Tocolysis can be done.

Infants born before 32 weeks of gestation, are at increased risk of HIV but may be unable to tolerate oral medication. Anti-retroviral therapy administered to the mother just before and during delivery will provide prophylaxis for the neonate. C

7.4. How should preterm prelabour rupture of the membranes be managed?

Where preterm prelabour rupture of the membranes occurs after 34 weeks of gestation, delivery should be expedited. D

A genital infection screen should be done and intravenous broad-spectrum antibiotics should be started.

Steroids should be administered in the usual way.

In untreated women, rupture of membranes for more than four hours is associated with a doubling of the risk of HIV transmission.

7.5. How should pre-labour rupture of the membranes at term be managed?

In case of prelabour rupture of the membranes at term, delivery should be expedited. D

Broad-spectrum intravenous antibiotics should be administered if there is evidence of genital infection or chorioamnionitis. D

There is a 2% incremental increase in transmission risk for every hour of ruptured membranes up to 24 hours.

7.6. How should prolonged pregnancy be managed?

For women on HAART with a plasma viral load of less than 50 copies/ml, the decision regarding induction of labour should be individualized. There is no contraindication for membrane sweeping or prostaglandins. D

7.7. What is the role of vaginal birth after caesarean section?

It may be considered for women taking HAART whose plasma viral load is less than 50 copies/ml. D

7.8. How should women diagnosed in late pregnancy but before the onset of labour be managed?

Women diagnosed with HIV late in pregnancy should have a rapid multidisciplinary team assessment and HAART should be commenced as soon as possible. D

7.9. How should women diagnosed with HIV during labour be managed?

For women who are HIV positive who are diagnosed during labour, urgent advice should be sought from the HIV physicians regarding HAART; delivery should be by caesarean section and, where possible, should be timed with respect to anti-retroviral administration. D

8. MANAGEMENT OF DELIVERY

8.1. How should caesarean section be managed?

a. If intravenous ZDV is indicated, the infusion should be started four hours before the caesarean section and should continue until the umbilical cord has been clamped. D

b. The surgical field should be kept as haemostatic as possible.

c. Care should be taken to try to avoid rupturing the membranes until the head is delivered.

d. The cord should be clamped as early as possible after delivery. D

e. A maternal sample for plasma viral load and CD4 lymphocyte count should be taken at delivery. D

f. Peripartum antibiotics should be administered.

8.2. How should planned vaginal delivery be managed?

a. Only women with a plasma viral load of less than 50 copies/ml should be offered a planned vaginal delivery. D

b. Invasive procedures such as foetal blood sampling and foetal scalp electrodes are contraindicated. D

c. If labour progress is normal, amniotomy should be avoided unless delivery is imminent. D

d. Amniotomy and oxytocin may be used for augmentation of labour. D

e. If instrumental delivery is indicated, the forceps is preferred to ventouse. D

9. POSTPARTUM CARE

9.1. What support should be given to women with respect to avoidance of breastfeeding?

Women who are HIV positive should be advised not to breastfeed. B

Women should be given advice about infant formula feeding.

Cabergoline one mg orally within 24 hours of birth is given to all women who are HIV positive to suppress lactation.

9.2. What contraceptive advice should be given?

All women who are HIV positive should receive advice about contraception in the immediatepostpartum period. D

Contraceptive counselling requires specialist advice.

9.3. What immunizations should be offered to the mother?

Measles, mumps, rubella and varicella zoster immunizations are given postpartum. D

Hepatitis B, pneumococcal and influenza vaccines are recommended for all people who are HIV positive (between October and March). These vaccines can be safely administered inpregnancy or postpartum.

10. CARE OF THE NEONATE

10.1 What antiretroviral therapy should be administered to the neonate?

All neonates born to HIV positive women should be treated with anti-retroviral therapy within four hours of birth. A

Most infants will be given ZDV monotherapy twice daily for four weeks.

HAART is given to infants at high risk of HIV infection.

Infants of untreated mothers.
Maternal viral load greater than 50 copies/ml.

The only licensed antiretroviral drug available for intravenous use in sick or preterm infants is ZDV. C

10.2. Should prophylaxis against PCP be administered to the neonate?

Prophylaxis against PCP is recommended only for infants born to mothers at high risk of transmission.

10.3. How and when should the infant be tested for HIV?

Infants should be tested at one day, six weeks and 12 weeks of age. If all these tests are negative and the baby is not being breastfed, the parents can be informed that the child is not HIV-infected. D

A confirmatory HIV antibody test is performed at around 18 months of age.

The gold-standard test for HIV in infants is HIV DNA polymerase chain reaction on peripheral blood lymphocytes.

11. PRE-PREGNANCY MANAGEMENT

For couples wishing to conceive where one or both partners is HIV positive, pre-pregnancy counselling should be done by appropriately trained health professional.

11.1. What interventions are there to minimize the risk of transmission between discordant couples at conception?

Couples who are serodiscordant for HIV infection and who choose to have sexual intercourse should be advised to use condoms. B

Consistent use of condoms is associated with an 80% reduction in transmission.

Serodiscordant couples where the female partner is HIV negative should be advised that assisted conception with either donor insemination or sperm washing is safer than timed unprotected intercourse. B

11.2. How should the health of the mother who is HIV positive and her foetus be optimized periconceptually?

Couples are recommended to delay conception until plasma viraemia is suppressed, prophylaxis against PCP is no longer required and opportunistic infections have been treated. D

Folate supplementation should be given. For women taking cotrimoxazole, higher dose folate (5 mg) should be administered. D

All women who are HIV positive are recommended to have yearly cervical cytology. B

69 Protocol Management of HIV in Pregnancy

ANTENATAL	
All pregnant patients are recommended to screen for HIV, hepatitis B, hepatitis C, syphilis and rubella.	
If patient declines screening of HIV at booking visit, then reason for decline should be explored and documented and again screening offered at 28 weeks.	
If patient is HIV negative but at high risk of acquiring infection then again screening is offered at 28 weeks.	
If patient is HIV positive then should be managed with multidisciplinary team.	
Viral load and CD4 lymphocyte count should be determined, and checked at each trimester, and at 36 weeks and then at delivery.	
HAART should be prescribed for women's health as soon as the HIV is diagnosed and continue even in postpartum period and if not required for women's health then for baby's health between 20–28 weeks.	
Genital infections should be screened and treated if asymptomatic.	
Immunization should be done for hepatitis B, pneumococcus and influenza.	
Women taking HAART should be screened for gestational diabetes and counselled for preterm delivery.	
Antenatal visit should be monthly till 28 weeks and then fortnightly till 36 weeks and weekly afterwards.	
Decision about mode of delivery should be made at 36 weeks in consultation with senior obstetrician and HIV physician.	
Mode of delivery will be decided according to viral load, if viral load of copies >50/ml then recommendation is caesarean delivery, vaginal delivery is permitted only in case of copies < 50/ml.	

INTRAPARTUM MANAGEMENT	
When HIV positive patient presents in labour, her viral load and decided mode about delivery should be reviewed.	
In case of caesarean delivery, zidovudine infusion should be started four hours before surgery. Field should be kept haemostatic and baby's head should be delivered with intact membranes.	
In case of vaginal delivery zidovudine infusion is started at onset of labour. Avoid rupturing of membranes and invasive monitoring. Use of forceps is preferable over vacuum if needed.	
Woman already on HAART will continue HAART postpartum.	
Paediatrician should receive the baby and baby should be given monotherapy or HAART depending on risk of infectivity.	
Testing of HIV in baby should be done at day one, six weeks, 12 weeks, then 18 month of age.	
Early bathing of baby is recommended.	
Breastfeeding is not recommended, formula feeding is advised.	
POSTPARTUM MANAGEMENT	
Continue HAART if patient requires.	
Effective contraception is advised (if family is complete then sterilization is offered. Otherwise barrier method is contraception of choice) or as advised by specialist.	

Guideline 70 Maternal Collapse in Pregnancy and the Puerperium

Adapted from Green-op Guideline No. 56

1. PURPOSE

To discuss the identification of women at increased risk of maternal collapse, causes of maternal collapse, to delineate the management of maternal collapse and to review maternal and neonatal outcomes.

2. BACKGROUND

Maternal collapse is defined as an acute event involving the cardiorespiratory systems and/or brain, resulting in a reduced or absent conscious level (and potentially death), at any stage in pregnancy and up to six weeks after delivery. It is such a rare event, with potentially devastating consequences. It is essential that caregivers are skilled in initial effective resuscitation techniques and are able to investigate and diagnose the cause of the collapse to allow appropriate, directed continuing management.

3. CLINICAL ISSUES

3.1. Can women at risk of impending collapse be identified early?

There should be early warning score chart for the recognition of the woman who is becoming critically ill. D

Antenatal care for women should include recognition of women at risk for collapse like with significant medical conditions and should include multidisciplinary team input with a pregnancy and delivery management plan in place **(Evidence level 4).**

3.2. What are the causes of maternal collapse?

The common reversible causes of maternal collapse in any woman are:

Haemorrhage Cardiac disease Eclampsia	Thromboembolism Drug toxicity/ overdose Sepsis	Amniotic fluid embolism Anaphylaxis Intracranial haemorrhage	Other causes as hypoglycaemia, metabolic and electrolyte disturbances

Causes of maternal collapse can also be grouped in the following manner.

Reversible cause		Cause in pregnancy
4 H's	Hypovolaemia	Bleeding (may be concealed) (obstetrics/ other) or relative hypovolaemia of dense spinal block; septic or neurogenic shock.
	Hypoxia	Pregnant patients can become hypoxic more quickly.
		Cardiac events: peripartum cardiomyopathy, myocardial infarction, aortic dissection, large-vessel aneurysms.
	Hypo/hyperkalaemia and other Electrolyte disturbances	No more likely.
	Hypothermia	No more likely.
4 T's	Thromboembolism	Amniotic fluid embolus, pulmonary embolus, air embolus, myocardial infarction.
	Toxicity	Local anaesthetic, magnesium, other.
	Tension pneumothorax	Following trauma/suicide attempt.
	Tamponade (cardiac)	Following trauma/suicide attempt.
Eclampsia and pre-eclampsia		Includes intracranial haemorrhage.

3.3. What is the optimal initial management of maternal collapse and how is it affected by maternal physiological changes of pregnancy?

It is essential that anyone involved in the resuscitation of pregnant women is aware of the physiological differences. This includes paramedics and emergency room staff. ✓

The standard approach to manage women with collapse is A, B, C with some modifications. After basic resuscitation if required urgent arrangement for transfer of women should be made. ✓

3.3.1. Tilt

Aortocaval compression significantly reduces cardiac output from 20 weeks of gestation onwards. In supine position after 20 weeks there is compression of aorta and inferior vena cava, which in turn reduces cardiac output by 30–40%. **(Evidence level 2+)**

From 20 weeks of gestation onwards, the pressure of the gravid uterus must be relieved from the inferior vena cava and aorta. C

A left lateral tilt of 15 degree on a firm surface will relieve aortocaval compression in the majority of pregnant women and still allow effective chest compressions to be performed. C

Left lateral tilt can be provided by someone kneeling on the right side of women and placing knee under the thorax of patient or alternatively using wedge for displacement of uterus manually **(Evidence level 2+)**.

3.3.2. Airway

In pregnancy, the airway is more vulnerable because of the increased risk of regurgitation and aspiration due to relaxing effect of progesterone on lower esophageal sphincter and raised intra abdominal pressure due to gravid uterus, for this reason it is important to clear and protect the airway as early as possible.

The airway should be protected as soon as possible by intubation with a cuffed endotracheal tube. ✓

Difficult intubation is more likelyin pregnancy due to weight gain, large size breasts and laryngeal oedema and should be carried out by skilled person. ✓

Intubation will protect airway, ensure proper oxygen supply and facilitate effective ventilation.

3.3.3. Breathing

Changes in lung function, diaphragmatic splinting and increased oxygen consumption make the pregnant woman become hypoxic more readily and make ventilation more difficult.

Supplemental oxygen should be administered as soon as possible. ✓

Bag and mask ventilation should be undertaken until intubation can be achieved. ✓

3.3.4. Circulation

The increased cardiac output and hyperdynamic circulation of pregnancy means that large volumes of blood can be lost rapidly, especially from the uterus, which receives 10% of the cardiac output at term, otherwise healthy women tolerate blood loss better and only become symptomatic after losing 35% of their circulation.

Aortocaval compression significantly reduces the efficacy of chest compressions during resuscitation as it further reduces cardiac output to 10% and aim of compression is to increase cardiac output **(Evidence level 2+)**.

In the absence of breathing despite a clear airway, chest compressions should be commencedimmediately. B

There should be an aggressive approach to volume. ✓

Two wide bore cannulas should be inserted as soon as possible. ✓

Compressions can be difficult due to obesity and tilt of women **(Evidence level 2++)**.

Compressions should be performed at a ratio of 30:2 ventilations unless the woman is intubated, in which case chest compressions and ventilations should be desynchronized with compressions being performed at a rate of 100/minute and ventilations at a rate of 10/minute. As after 20 weeks, compressions are not very effective, early recourse to delivery of foetus and placenta if CPR is not effective **(Evidence level 2 ++)**.

Abdominal ultrasound by a skilled operator can assist in the diagnosis of concealed haemorrhage. C

The same defibrillation energy levels should be used as in the nonpregnant patient. B

3.3.5. Drugs

There should normally be no alteration in drugs or doses. ✓

Common, reversible causes of maternal cardiopulmonary arrest should be considered throughout the resuscitation process. D

Resuscitation efforts should be continued until a decision is taken by the consultant obstetricianand consultant anaesthetist in consensus with the cardiac arrest team. ✓

3.4. When, where and how should perimortem caesarean section be performed?

If there is no response to correctly performed CPR within four minutes of maternal collapse or if resuscitation is continued beyond this in women beyond 20 weeks of gestation, delivery should be undertaken to assist maternal resuscitation. This should be achieved within five minutes of the collapse as hypoxia occurs early in pregnant women leading to brain death within 4–6 minutes. D

Delivery of the baby and placenta improves venous return and cardiac output; facilitates chest compressions and makes ventilation easier **(Evidence level 4)**.

Perimortem caesarean section should be considered a resuscitative procedure to be performed primarily in the interest of maternal, not foetal, survival.

Perimortem caesarean section should not be delayed by moving the woman—it should be performed where resuscitation is taking place.	✓
The operator should use the incision that will facilitate the most rapid access. The incision which gives most rapid access is midline abdominal and classical uterine incision but operator should use approach which is comfortable for operator.	✓
A perimortem caesarean section tray should be available on the resuscitation trolley in all areas where maternal collapse may occur, including the accident and emergency department.	✓

3.5. What does the continuing management consist of?

Senior staff with appropriate experience should be involved at an early stage.	✓
Transfer should be supervised by an adequately skilled team with appropriate equipment.	✓

3.5.1. Haemorrhage

The management of PPH is given in PPH guideline.	
In the case of maternal collapse secondary to antepartum haemorrhage, the foetus and placenta should be delivered promptly to allow control of the haemorrhage.	✓
In the case of massive placental abruption, caesarean section may occasionally be indicated even if the foetus is dead to allow rapid control of the haemorrhage.	✓

3.5.2. Venous thromboembolism

Appropriate use of thromboprophylaxis and thrombolytic therapy in the form of heparin is required.

3.5.3. Amniotic fluid embolism

The management of amniotic fluid embolismis supportive rather than specific, as there is no proven effective therapy.	✓

Early involvement of senior experienced staff, including obstetrician, anaesthetist, haematologist and intensivist, is essential to optimize outcome. ✓

Coagulopathy needs early, aggressive treatment, including aggressive use of fresh frozen plasma. ✓

3.5.4. Cardiac disease

After successful resuscitation, cardiac cases should be managed, by an expert cardiology team.	✓

3.5.5. Sepsis

Septic shock should be managed according to the sepsis guidelines.

A multidisciplinary team approach is required including midwives, consultant obstetricians, consultant anaesthetists, consultant haematologists, consultant intensivists and consultant microbiologists. The following 'care bundle' should be applied immediately or within six hours, and has been shown to significantly improve survival rates:

1. Measure serum lactate. Serum lactate rises in sepsis due to anaerobic metabolism. Lactate is a useful method of determining prognosis with those who have a level greater than 4 mmol/L having a mortality of 40% and those with a level of less than 2 mmol/L have a mortality of less than 15%.
2. Obtain blood cultures/culture swabs prior to antibiotic administration.
3. Administer broad-spectrum antibiotic(s) within the first hour of recognition of severe sepsis and septic shock according to local protocol
4. In the event of hypotension and/or lactate >4 mmol/l:
   a. Deliver an initial minimum of 20 ml/kg of crystalloid/colloid
   b. Once adequate volume replacement has been achieved, a vasopressor (norepinephrine, epinephrine) and/or an inotrope (e.g. dobutamine) may be used to maintain mean arterialpressure over 65 mmHg.

Further management consists of:

1. In the event of hypotension despite fluid resuscitation (septic shock) and/or lactate over 4 mmol/l:

a. Achieve a central venous pressure of at least 8 mmHg (or over 12 mmHg if the woman is mechanically ventilated) with aggressive fluid replacement.

b. Consider steroids.

2. Maintain oxygen saturation with facial oxygen. Consider transfusion if haemoglobin is below 7 g/dl.

3.5.6. Drug overdose/toxicity

In obstetric practice, the two main drugs that can give rise to overdose or toxic problems are magnesium sulphate and local anaesthetic agents.

Magnesium sulphate

The antidote to magnesium toxicity is 10 ml of 10% calcium gluconate given by slow intravenous injection.

Local anaesthetic agents

If local anaesthetic toxicity is suspected, stop injecting immediately. ✓

Lipid rescue should be used in cases of collapse secondary to local anaesthetic toxicity. C

Intralipid 20% should be available in all maternity units. Manage arrhythmias as usual, recognizing that they may be very refractory to treatment. ✓

3.5.7. Eclampsia

Should be managed according to protocol of eclampsia given in guideline of management of severe preeclampsia and eclampsia.

3.5.8. Intracranial haemorrhage

Expert neuroradiology is required to establish an accurate diagnosis. Management is the same as in the nonpregnant state, although delivery may be necessary to facilitate this. The appropriate experts should be involved at the earliest opportunity.

3.5.9. Anaphylaxis

In cases of anaphylaxis, all potential causative agents should be removed, and the A, B, C, D, E approach followed. A

The definitive treatment for anaphylaxis is 500 micrograms (0.5 ml) of 1:1000 adrenaline intramuscularly. **Please note this dose is for intramuscular use only.** A

Adrenaline treatment can be repeated after five minutes if there is no effect.

Adjuvant therapy consists of chlopheniramine 10 mg and hydrocortisone 200 mg, both can be given intramuscularly or slow intravenously.

3.6. Who should be on the team?

In addition to the general arrest team, there should be a senior midwife, an obstetrician and an obstetric anaesthetist included in the team in cases of maternal collapse. ✓

If the maternity unit is an integral part of a general hospital, the maternal cardiopulmonary resuscitation team should be the hospital cardiopulmonary arrest team with the addition of:

A senior midwife.

The most senior resident obstetrician.

A resident anaesthetist who has recognized skills in obstetric anaesthesia.

The consultant obstetrician and consultant obstetric anaesthetist should be summoned at the time of the cardiopulmonary arrest call. ✓

The neonatal team should be called early if delivery is likely (antepartum collapse over 22 weeks of gestation). ✓

Where the woman survives, a consultant intensivist should be involved as soon as possible. ✓

4. DOCUMENTATION

Accurate documentation in all cases of maternal collapse, whether or not resuscitation is successful, is essential. ✓

Protocol Maternal Collapse in Pregnancy and the Puerperium

71

This is an obstetrical emergency and its management includes understanding of physiological changes occurring during pregnancy along with risk factors of collapse.	
Call for help.	
Team approach (multidisciplinary) is required to carry out resuscitation and assessment side by side.	
Tilt patient on left side by 15 degrees if she is more than 20 weeks pregnant by placing wedge on right side to avoid aortocaval compression.	
Secure and maintain airway of patient by head tilt and jaw thrust manoeuvre and intubation, intubation can be difficult in pregnant women so should be carried out by skilled person as it provides effective ventilation.	
100% oxygen should be given by face mask and bag.	
If patient is not breathing, start chest compression, ratio of chest compression with ventilation 30:2, continue till advance life support approaches.	
Save two I/V lines with 18 gauge cannula and send investigations including CBC, clotting profile, liver function tests, renal function tests, electrolytes, blood sugar random, blood cross match and arterial blood gases.	
Order blood and blood products.	
Catheterize the patient.	
Start fluid resuscitation.	
Assess the cause of collapse and treat it accordingly.	

Continue CPR for four minutes if no response, then immediately do postmortem caesarean section at the same place doing CPR without anaesthesia.	
Baby should be handed over to paediatrician.	
If the patient responds after that, then shift patient to theatre, anaesthetise her and complete caesarean section.	
If resuscitation is successful then shift patient to ICU and search for cause of collapse and treat it.	
Otherwise resuscitation efforts should be continued until a decision is taken by the consultant obstetrician, anaesthetist and the cardiac arrest team.	

Guideline 72
Obstetric Cholestasis

Adapted from Green Top Guideline No. 43, April 2011

1. PURPOSE

To identify the maternal and foetal risks of obstetric cholestasis.

To discuss management options for obstetric cholestasis.

2. BACKGROUND

It is a multifactorial condition of pregnancy characterised by intense pruritus and abnormal liver function test in the absence of skin rash. Both pruritus and abnormal liver function test are not due to any other cause and remit following delivery. Pruritus on palms and soles of feet are more suggestive.

It affects 0.7% of pregnancies in multi ethnic population and 1.2–1.5% pregnancies in Indian or Pakistani and people of asian origin.

3. DIAGNOSIS

Diagnosis is made on the basis of symptoms, signs and investigations. Other causes of liver dysfunction and pruritus should also be excluded.

Symptoms: Pruritus, usually worse at night, is widespread and may involve palms and soles. Other symptoms of cholestasis include dark urine and pale stools.

Ask regarding personal and family history of obstetric cholestasis, multiple pregnancy, gallstones and carriers of hepatitis. C

Anorexia and insomnia may be present.

Sign: No skin rash but jaundice can be present.

Investigations

Specific for obstetric cholestasis	Rule out other differential diagnosis
Liver function test. Bile salts only when LFTs persistently remain normal.	Viral screening of hepatitis A, B, C, Epstein-Barr virus, cytomegalovirus. Autoimmune screening for chronic active hepatitis and primary biliary cirrhosis. Liver ultrasound.

Pre-eclampsia and acute fatty liver of pregnancy are pregnancy specific differentials of abnormal liver function test. Other differentials include viral hepatitis, primary biliary cirrhosis, chronic active hepatitis and gall stones.

In clinical practice abnormalities in transaminases, gama glutamyl transferase, bilirubin and/or bile salts are considered sufficient to support the diagnosis of obstetric cholestasis.

Bilirubin is only increased infrequently and most women will have increased levels of one or more of the three other liver function tests.

LFTs should be carried out 1–2 weekly in patients with persistent pruritus as they may take days to weeks to become abnormal after pruritus.

Isolated elevation of bile salts is rare and should not be carried out routinely, only done in patients with persistently normal LFTs.

In pregnancy, bilirubin level does not show much change but SGPT and SGOT reduces by 20%, alkaline phosphatase increases.

Pregnancy specific ranges of LFTs should be used.	C
Other causes of itching and of liver dysfunction should be excluded.	C
Postnatal resolution of pruritus and LFTs should be confirmed.	C
Women with persistent pruritus and normal biochemistry should have LFTs repeated every 1–2 weekly.	C

1. What is the risk of stillbirth in pregnancy complicated by obstetric cholestasis?

In hospital settings, the risk of stillbirth in women with obstetric cholestasis as compared to general population is not determined but is likely to be small. B

2. What additional risk is associated in pregnancy complicated with obstetric complication?

Premature birth both spontaneous and iatrogenic.	B
Meconium stained liquor.	B
Foetal distress.	B
Caesarean section.	B
PPH.	B

3. Can foetal death be predicted and prevented?

Delivery decision should not be based on the degree of abnormality of biochemical test, as current data are not robust enough to demonstrate or exclude correlation with intrauterine death and abnormal liver function test of raised bile salts. B

No specific foetal monitoring modality for the prediction of foetal death can be recommended. C

Ultrasound is not a reliable method for preventing foetal death in obstetric cholestasis. B

Continuous foetal monitoring should be offered in labour. ✓

IUD has no evidence of placental insufficiency and is usually sudden, seems to be due to sudden anoxia. **(Evidence level 2+)**.

4. What treatment if any should be used to treat obstetric cholestasis and what benefit can be expected?

Topical emollients are safe but their efficacy is unknown. C

It only improves pruritus.

Systemic treatment as cholestyramine may improve pruritus but exacerbates vitamin K deficiency and is not subjected to any randomized controlled trials.

Antihistamines only improve pruritus by inducing sleep.

Adenosyl methionine

There is insufficient evidence to show whether S adenosyl methionine is effective for either control of maternal symptoms or for improving foetal outcomes.

Ursodeoxycholic acid A

Women should be aware of the lack of data to show any improvement in the pruritus or protection against foetal death. ✓

Dexamethasone

It should not be first line therapy for the treatment of obstetric cholestasis, nor should it be used outside of an RCT without a thorough consultation with the women. B

Some studies show adverse foetal and neonatal neurological effects after the use of Dexamethasone for obstetric cholestasis.

5. What is the role of vitamin K?

There is sparse data regarding use of vitamin K in antenatal period but its use is beneficial as obstetric cholestasis results in fat malabsorption which reduces absorption of fat soluble vitamin including vitamin K, decreases formation of factor II, VII, IX and X, so 10 mg vitamin K in antenatal period is beneficial in reducing PPH, foetal and neonatal bleeding **(Evidence level 4).**

Vitamin K is associated with haemolytic disease, hyperbilirubinaemia and kernicterus in neonates but in low doses it is rare **(Evidence level 3).**

Post-natal vitamin K must be offered to babies in a routine manner.

6. How should obstetric cholestasis be monitored?

Measure LFTs weekly until delivery. ✓

Postnatal LFTs should be deferred for at least 10 days as LFTs increase in first 10 days after delivery so should be carried out after that time. C

7. Should women with obstetric cholestasis be offered elective early delivery?

The discussion regarding delivery should be carried out with women at 37 weeks. She should be told that delivery at this gestation has increase chances of perinatal morbidity but if there is severe biochemical derangement then it strongly supports delivery at 37 weeks. ✓ and B

Women should be informed of inability to predict stillbirth if pregnancy continues. ✓

As there is no time of stillbirth in obstetric cholestasis so after reaching 37 weeks its reasonable to offer delivery as term has achieved and stillbirth beyond it can be avoided by delivery at 37 weeks **(Evidence level 2 ++)**.

8. What follow up should be offered to women who have had pregnancy affected by obstetric cholestasis?

Women should be followed to ensure that LFTs have returned to normal and to provide appropriate counselling.

Reassure women regarding no long term sequelae of obstetric cholestasis on women and baby, the high recurrence rate, contraceptive advice (avoid oestrogen containing methods) and increase chances of obstetric cholestasis in family members.

73 Protocol Obstetric Cholestasis

DESIRED PATIENT OUTCOMES	
To maintain pregnancy, promote optimal well being of mother and baby.	
ASSESSMENT	
History: Intense pruritus especially on palms and soles of feet, without rash, usually occurring at night. Rule out dark urine and pale stools.	
Examination: No skin rash but jaundice can be present.	
INVESTIGATIONS	
LFTs and if LFTs persistently remain normal than bile salts.	
To exclude other causes, ultrasound of liver, viral screening for hepatitis A, B, C, Epstein Barr and cytomegalovirus and autoimmune screening are recommended.	
PATIENT CARE	
No test can predict foetal stillbirth.	
Admission is optional.	
CTG on alternate day.	
Monitor LFTs weekly in antenatal period.	
Steroid cover Injection Betamethasone 12 mg two doses intramuscular, 24 hours apart.	
Neonatal facility should be present in hospital.	
PATIENT EDUCATION	
Risk of stillbirth is undetermined but less in hospital settings.	

There is no way to predict and prevent stillbirth in obstetric cholestasis. No test including ultrasound and CTG can predict stillbirth.	
Other complications of obstetric cholestasis are preterm delivery, meconium stained liquor, foetal distress, increased probability of C-section and PPH.	
Counsel patient that obstetrics cholestasis has no long term effect on mother and neonate.	
It has high recurrence rate (45–90%).	
Avoid use of oestrogen containing contraception.	
PATIENT INSTRUCTION	
Note foetal movements daily.	
PATIENT TREATMENT	
Topical emollients for pruritus.	
Ursodeoxycholic acid improves pruritus and improves LFTs.	
Tab vitamin K 10 mg daily in antenatal period.	
Though there is no evidence that delivery at 37 weeks will improve foetal outcome but in view of increased probability of foetal distress and meconium, it is recommended that time of delivery and possible complications should be discussed in detail with the couple and delivery should be considered at 37 weeks.	
Continuous foetal heart rate monitoring, during labour.	
Routine vitamin K should be given to neonate at birth.	
PATIENT'S FOLLOW UP	
Repeat LFTs after six weeks	
If required, refer patient to medical physician.	
DOCUMENTATION	
Gestational age, any meconium stained liquor, steroid given, time and mode of delivery and APGAR score of baby.	

74 Guideline Operative Vaginal Delivery

Adapted from Green-top Guideline No. 26, July 2011

1. PURPOSE

The aim of this guideline is to provide up-to-date information on the use of forceps and vacuum extractor, to expedite delivery with a minimum of maternal or neonatal morbidity.

2. BACKGROUND

There has been increasing awareness of the potential for morbidity for both the mother and the baby with operative vaginal delivery. The increased risk of neonatal morbidity in relation to operative vaginal delivery is long established, although with careful practice, over all rates of morbidity are low.

3. PREPARATION FOR OPERATIVE VAGINAL DELIVERY

3.1. Can operative vaginal delivery be avoided?

Factors which reduce the chances of operative vaginal delivery	
Support during labour.	A
Upright or lateral position during labour.	A
Avoidance of epidural analgesia.	A

Delayed pushing in primiparous women with an epidural can reduce the need for rotational and midcavity deliveries. A

3.2. How should operative vaginal delivery be classified?

A standard classification of operative vaginal delivery should be used. D

3.2.1. Outlet

Foetal scalp visible without separating the labia.

Foetal skull has reached the pelvic floor.

Sagittal suture is in the anterio-posterior diameter or right or left occiput anterior or posterior position (rotation does not exceed 45°).

Foetal head is at or on the perineum.

3.2.2. Low

Leading point of the skull (not caput) is at station plus 2 cm or more and not on the pelvic floor.

3.2.3. Mid

Foetal head is no more than 1/5th palpable per abdomen.

Leading point of the skull is between 0–2 station (below Ischial spines but above +2 station).

Should only be performed by experienced person with minimal morbidity to mother and baby.

3.2.4. High

Operative vaginal delivery is not recommended.

Head is 2/5th or more palpable abdominally.

Presenting part is above the level of the ischial spines vaginally.

3.3. When should operative vaginal delivery be offered?

Indications for operative vaginal delivery

Foetal

Foetal distress.

Maternal

1. To shorten the second stage of labour on medical conditions (e.g. cardiac disease Class III or IV, hypertensive crises, myasthenia gravis, spinal cord injury patients at risk of autonomic dysreflexia, proliferative retinopathy).
2. Inadequate progress.
3. Maternal exhaustion.

A vacuum extractor should not be used at gestation of less than 34 weeks and should be used with caution between 34–36 weeks. At less than 36 weeks, there is risk of subgaleal and intracranial haemorrhage. D

3.4. What are the essential conditions for safe operative vaginal delivery?

Safe operative vaginal delivery requires a careful assessment of the clinical situation, clear communication with the mother and healthcare personnel and expertise in the chosen procedure. D

Prerequisites for operative vaginal delivery

Full abdominal and vaginal examination

Head is ≤1/5th palpable per abdomen.

Vertex presentation.

Cervix is fully dilated and the membranes ruptured.

Exact position of the head should be known.

Assessment of caput and moulding.

Pelvis should be adequate, irreducible moulding may indicate cephalo pelvic disproportion.

Preparation of mother

Clear explanation should be given and informed consent obtained.

Appropriate analgesia, regional block or pudendal block may be appropriate, particularly in case of urgent delivery.

Maternal bladder should be empty.

Aseptic technique.

Preparation of staff

Operator must have the knowledge, experience and skills necessary.

Adequate facilities are available (appropriate equipment, bed, and lighting).

Back-up plan in place in case of failure to deliver. When conducting mid-cavity delivery, theatre staff should be immediately available to allow a caesarean section to be performed without delay (less than 30 minutes).

A senior obstetrician competent in performing mid-cavity delivery should be present if a junior trainee is performing the delivery.

Anticipation of complications that may arise (e.g. shoulder dystocia, postpartum haemorrhage).

Paediatrician should be present.

3.5. What type of consent is required?

Women should be informed in the antenatal period about operative vaginal delivery, especially during their first pregnancy.

For deliveries in the delivery room, verbal consent should be obtained before an operative vaginal delivery and the discussion documented in the notes. If circumstances allow, written consent may also be obtained.

Written consent should be obtained for a trial of operative vaginal delivery in theatre.

4. PERFORMING OPERATIVE VAGINAL DELIVERY

4.1. Who should perform operative vaginal delivery?

An operative vaginal delivery should be performed by an operator who has the knowledge, experience and skills necessary to assess and to use the instruments and manage complications that may arise. D

Obstetricians should achieve experience in spontaneous vertex delivery before commencing training in operative vaginal delivery.

Obstetric trainees should receive appropriate training in operative vaginal delivery. Competency should be achieved before conducting unsupervised deliveries and should be monitored regularly thereafter.

4.2. Where should operative vaginal delivery take place?

Operative vaginal births that have a higher risk of failure should be considered a trial and conducted in a place where immediate recourse to caesarean section can be undertaken. C

Higher rates of failure are associated with:

Maternal body mass index over 30.

Estimated foetal weight over 4000 g or clinically big baby.

Occipito-posterior position.

Mid-cavity delivery or when 1/5th of the head palpable per abdomen.

4.3. What instruments should be used for operative vaginal delivery?

The operator should choose the instrument most appropriate to the clinical circumstances and their level of skill. Forceps and vacuum extraction are associated with different benefits and risks. Failed delivery with selected instrument is more likely with vacuum extraction. A

The options available for rotational delivery include Keilland's forceps, manual rotation followed by direct traction forceps or rotational vacuum extraction. Rotational deliveries should be performed, by experienced operators, with the choice depending on the expertise of the individual operator.

There is insufficient evidence to favour either a rapid (over two minutes) or a stepwise increment in negative pressure with vacuum extraction.

4.4. When should operative vaginal delivery be abandoned?

Operative vaginal delivery should be abandoned where there is no evidence of progressive descent with moderate traction during each contraction or where delivery is not imminent following three contractions of a correctly applied instrument by an experienced operator. B

Adverse outcomes, including unsuccessful forceps or vacuum delivery, should trigger an incident report as part of effective risk management processes.

4.5. Is there a place for sequential use of instruments?

The use of sequential instruments is associated with an increased risk of trauma to the infant; however, the operator must balance the risks of a caesarean section following failed vacuum extraction with the risks of forceps delivery following failed vacuum extraction. B

Obstetricians should be aware of increased neonatal morbidity with failed operative vaginal delivery and/or sequential use of instruments and should inform the neonatologist when this occurs to ensure appropriate management of the baby.

4.6. What is the role of episiotomy for operative vaginal delivery?

Episiotomy decision should be on individualized basis and there is no need to give episiotomy in every case of operative vaginal delivery. B

4.7. Should prophylactic antibiotics be given?

There is no need of prophylactic antibiotic. A

Good standards of hygiene and aseptic techniques are recommended.

5.1. Should thromboprophylaxis be given?

Women should be reassessed after an operative vaginal delivery for risk factors for venousthromboembolism, if appropriate thromboprophylaxis should be prescribed. D

5.2. What analgesia should be given after delivery?

Regular paracetamol and diclofenac should be offered after an operative vaginal delivery in the absence of contraindications.

5.3. What precautions should be taken for care of the bladder after delivery?

The timing and volume of the first void urine should be monitored and documented. C

A post-void residual should be measured if retention is suspected.

Physiotherapy should be offered to women to avoid urinary incontinence after operative vaginal delivery. A

5.4. How can we reduce psychological morbidity for the mother?

There is no evidence to support the use of midwife-led debriefing in reducing maternal depression following operative vaginal delivery.	A

The woman should be reviewed prior to hospital discharge to discuss the indication for operative delivery, management of any complications and the prognosis for future deliveries. Best practice would be for the woman to be reviewed by the obstetrician who conducted the delivery.	

5.5. How should we advise women for future deliveries?

Women should be encouraged to aim for a spontaneous vaginal delivery in a subsequent pregnancy, as there is a high probability of success. B

Care should be individualized for women who have sustained a third or fourth degree perineal tear.

Protocol
Operative Vaginal Delivery 75

PREREQUISITES	
Preparation of mother	
Informed consent.	
Bladder should be emptied.	
Adequate analgesia.	
Aseptic technique.	
Preparation of staff	
Experienced operator.	
Adequate facilities available (equipment, bed, light).	
Backup facility of theatre in cases of failed delivery.	
Anticipation of complications (PPH, shoulder dystocia).	
Paediatrician should be present.	
Abdominal and vaginal examination	
Head < 1/5th palpable abdominally.	
Vertex presentation.	
Cervix fully dilated.	
Membranes ruptured.	
Position of head should be known.	
Assess caput and moulding.	
Adequate pelvis.	

INDICATIONS OF OPERATIVE VAGINAL DELIVERY	
Foetal	
Presumed foetal distress.	

To shorten second stage in certain conditions such as class III and IV cardiac disease. Hypertensive crisis. Myasthenia gravis. Spinal cord injury. Proliferative retinopathy. Inadequate progress, in primagravida two hours without regional anaesthesia and three hours with regional anaesthesia, in multigravida one hour without regional anaesthesia and two hours with regional anaesthesia.	
Maternal **Contraindications** Vacuum extractor should not be used in: ○ Face presentation. ○ Gestational age <34 weeks. ○ Breech presentation. Vacuum and forceps are contraindicated before full dilatation of cervix.	
Method of operative delivery It should be done according to checklist of forceps and vacuum delivery.	
Postnatal care Care of episiotomy. Regular paracetamol or diclofenac sodium to be given in absence of contraindications. If indicated, thromboprophylaxis should be given.	

Guideline
Preterm Premature Rupture of Membranes 76

Adapted from Green-top Guideline No. 44, October 2010

1. PURPOSE

The aim of this guideline is to make recommendations relating to the diagnosis, investigation and management of Preterm Prelabour Rupture of Membranes (PPROM). The guideline also evaluates the role of prophylactic antibiotic, steroid cover, optimum time of delivery and prediction of intrauterine foetal infection.

2. BACKGROUND

PPROM complicates only 2% of pregnancies but is associated with 40% of preterm deliveries and can result in significant neonatal morbidity and mortality. The three causes of neonatal death associated with PPROM are prematurity, sepsis and pulmonary hypoplasia. Women with intrauterine infection deliver earlier than non-infected women and infants born with sepsis have mortality four times higher than those without sepsis.

3. HOW IS THE DIAGNOSIS OF PPROM BEST ACHIEVED?

Diagnosis is achieved by: B

Maternal history (gush of fluid from vagina).

Speculum examination (pool of fluid seen).

Ultrasound in some cases (decrease amount of liquor).

A range of tests have been used to confirm membrane rupture, the most widely used is Nitrazine test, which detects PH change with sensitivity of 90%. **(Evidence level 2 b).**

Digital vaginal examination should be avoided because micro-organisms may be transported from the vagina into cervix leading to intrauterine infection, prostaglandin release and preterm labour. **(Evidence level 2 b).**

Diagnostic signs for chorioamnionitis
Offensive vaginal discharge.
Maternal tachycardia.
Maternal pyrexia.
Uterine tenderness.
Foetal tachycardia.
Leucocytosis.

3.1. What antenatal tests should be performed?

Women should be observed for signs of chorioamnionitis. ✓

Weekly high vaginal swab need not be performed. ✓

It is not necessary to carry out weekly maternal full blood count or C-reactive protein because the sensitivity of these tests in the detection of intrauterine infection is low. ✓

Cardiotocography is useful especially in detecting foetal tachycardia in case of chorioamnionitis. Biophysical profile score and Doppler velocity meter can be carried out, but women should be informed that these tests are of limited value in predicting foetal well being. B

3.2. What is the role of amniocentesis?

Intrauterine infections with positive amniotic fluid cultures, is found in 36% of women with PPROM. Most infections are subclinical associated with risks of preterm delivery, neonatal sepsis, respiratory distress, chronic lung disease, periventricular leukomalacia, intraventricular haemorrhage and cerebral palsy. **(Evidence level 2 a)**

Amniocentesis detects subclinical infection before the onset of maternal signs of chorioamnionitis and before the onset of foetal sepsis allowing appropriate intervention but there is not sufficient evidence to carry out amniocentesis to rule out subclinical intrauterine infections. **(Evidence level 2 a)**B

4. MANAGEMENT

4.1. Treatment

4.1.1 Are prophylactic antibiotics recommended?

Benefits of Antibiotic
Prolong pregnancy.
Reduce chances of chorioamnionitis.
Reduction in neonatal infection.
Reduction in abnormal cerebral ultrasound of neonate.

Erythromycin should be given for 10 days following the diagnosis of PPROM. A

4.1.2 What is the role of antenatal corticosteroids?

Antenatal corticosteroids should be given in women with PPROM between 24 and 34 weeks of gestation. A

4.1.3 Should tocolytic agents be used?

It is not recommended as it does not significantly improve perinatal outcome. A

In the absence of clear evidence that tocolysis improves neonatal outcome following PPROM, it is reasonable not to use it. Additionally, with PPROM in the presence of uterine contractions, it is possible that tocolysis could have adverse effects, such as delaying delivery from an infected environment, since there is an association between intrauterine infection, prostaglandin and cytokine release and delivery.

4.2. What is the appropriate time to deliver the baby?

Delivery should be considered at 34 weeks of gestation. While during expectant management, women should be informed regarding increase risk of chorioamnionitis and decrease risk of respiratory problems in neonates.	B

4.3. Can the woman be monitored at home?

It is recommended to stay in hospital for at least 48 hours before deciding other the patient can go home or not. At home regular temperature recording is advised after every 4–8 hours **(Evidence level 3).**

4.4. Should amnioinfusion in labour be carried out?

It is not recommended to carry out amnioinfusion in labour in women with PPROM.	A

4.5. What is the role of transabdominal amnioinfusion in the prevention of pulmonary hypoplasia?

There is insufficient evidence to recommend amnioinfusion in very preterm PPROM as a method to prevent pulmonary hypoplasia.

4.6. What is the role of fibrin glue in the sealing of chorioamniotic membrane to prevent pulmonary hypoplasia?

There is insufficient evidence to recommend fibrin sealants as routine treatment for second trimester oligohydramnios caused by PPROM.	B

Protocol 77
Management of PPROM

Preterm, Premature Rupture of Membranes (PPROM)

DESIRED PATIENT OUTCOMES	
To maintain pregnancy and promote optimal well being of mother and foetus.	
ASSESSMENT: Confirm the diagnosis.	
HISTORY	
Examination Maternal pulse and temperature.	
Uterine tenderness, uterine contractions, FHR.	
Amniotic fluid (amount, colour, odour).	
Investigations Send CBC, C-reactive protein, urine complete examination, High vaginal swab for culture and sensitivity, and microscopy for foetal cells (Nile blue test).	
Obstetrical USG for AFI and biophysical profile.	
PATIENT CARE	
Counsel patient regarding prognosis, labour, and mode of delivery.	
Ensure availability of neonatal facilities or in utero transfer.	
Daily foetal monitoring and non-stress test.	
Encourage good hygiene.	
Give antibiotics (Tab. erythromycin 250 mg QID).	
Give steroids (Injection betamethasone or dexamethasone 12 mg I/M, two doses 24 hours apart).	
Restrict patient's mobility.	
Assessment of amniotic fluid (amount, colour and odour) daily.	

	Watch for signs of chorioamnionitis (pulse, temp).	
	Amniotic fluid index, TLC and C-reactive protein.	
	CTG, Biophysical Profile (BPP)> 34 weeks gestation.	
	Decision about mode and time of delivery.	
WARNING SIGNS AND REPORTABLE CONDITIONS		
	Signs of infection (elevated temperature/maternal pulse).	
	Change in the amount, colour and/or odor of amniotic fluid.	
	Chills, flu-like symptoms, general malaise.	
	Abdominal tenderness, contractions or vaginal bleeding.	
	Foetal heart rate baseline changes decreased long term variability, presence of decelerations and/or a non-reactive NST. Decrease in or absence of foetal activity.	
	Decreased foetal movements.	
TIMING OF DELIVERY		
a.	Sign of chorioamnionitis.	
b.	Duration of pregnancy beyond 34 weeks.	
DOCUMENTATION		
	Gestational age, signs of chorioamnionitis, steroid cover, time and mode of delivery.	

References:

ACOG Guideline

RCOG Guideline

Guideline 78
Reduced Foetal Movements

Adapted from Green Top Guideline Number 57

1. PURPOSE

The purpose of this guideline is management of women with reduced foetal movements during pregnancy.

2. BACKGROUND

Foetal movements have been defined as any discrete kick, flutter, swish or roll.

Reduced or absent foetal movement may be warning signs of impending foetal death.

55% of women who had stillbirth felt a reduction in foetal movements prior to diagnosis.

3. WHAT ARE CONSIDERED NORMAL FOETAL MOVEMENTS DURING PREGNANCY?

Most women perceive foetal movements as early as 16 weeks and as late as 20 weeks.

The number of movements tends to increase upto 32nd week of pregnancy, after which the frequency plateaus until the onset of labour. However the type of foetal movement may change in late third trimester. **(Evidence level 2)**

By term on an average there are about 31 movements in one hour and longest period between movements varies from 50 to 75 minutes. **(Evidence level 2)**

The afternoon and evening period is usually the peak time of foetal movements. foetal movements are usually absent during sleep cycle, which occur regularly throughout day and night and usually last for 20 to 40 minutes. These sleep cycles rarely exceed 90 minutes in the normal healthy foetus.

(Evidence level 2)

There is no universally agreed definition of reduced foetal movements.

Most women are aware of foetal movements by 20th week of gestation.	C
Clinicians should be aware that although foetal movements tend to plateau at 32 weeks of gestation, there is no reduction in frequency of foetal movements in the late third trimester.	B

4. WHAT ARE THE FACTORS WHICH INFLUENCE A WOMAN'S PERCEPTION OF FOETAL ACTIVITY?

Before 28 weeks of gestation, an anteriorly placed placenta may decrease a woman's perception of foetal movements.	**(Evidence level 2-)**
Sedating drugs, which cross the placenta, have transient effect on foetal movements.	**(Evidence level 3)**
From 30 weeks onward, the level of carbon dioxide in maternal blood influences foetal respiratory movements and occurs in smokers.	
Corticosteroids decrease foetal movements and heart rate variability detected by CTG over the two days following administration.	**(Evidence level 2-)**
Foetuses with major malformation are associated with decrease foetal movements, due to abnormalities of CNS, muscular dysfunction or skeletal abnormalities.	
Foetal presentation has no effect on perception of movement.	**(Evidence level 2+)**
Foetal position might influence maternal perception, 80% of foetal spines lay anteriorly in women who are unable to perceive foetal movements	**(Evidence level 2-)**
Women perceive most foetal movement while lying down.	
Busy women usually do not perceive movements.	

Several studies record increase in foetal movements after increased glucose concentration in maternal blood.	

Women should be advised of the need to be aware of foetal movements up to and including the onset of labour and should report any decrease or cessation of foetal movements to their maternity unit.

5. HOW CAN FOETAL MOVEMENTS BE ASSESSED?

By subjective maternal perception of foetal movements. C

6. SHOULD FOETAL MOVEMENTS BE COUNTED ROUTINELY IN A FORMAL MANNER?

There is insufficient evidence to recommend formal foetal movement counting using specified alarm limits. B

Women should be advised to be aware of their baby's individual pattern of movements. If they are concerned about the reduction or cessation of foetal movements after 28 weeks, they should immediately contact their doctor. C

If woman are unsure whether movements are reduced after 28 weeks of gestation, they should be advised to lie on their left side and focus on foetal movements for two hoursi. If they do not feel 10 or more discrete movements in two hours, they should contact their doctor immediately. C

7. HOW CAN YOU MANAGE REDUCED FOETAL MOVEMENTS?

7.1. What should be included in clinical history?

A relevant history should be taken to assess the woman's risk factor for stillbirth and FGR. B

The clinician should be aware of the potential association of decreased foetal movements with key risk factors such as FGR, small for gestational age foetus, placental insufficiency and congenital abnormality.

History
Maternal age to rule out extreme of maternal age.
Parity as primi parity is risk factor.
Duration of reduced foetal movements.
Any previous history of reduced foetal movements.
Known IUGR or SGA.
Hypertension.
Diabetes.
Smoking.
Congenital malformation.
Race.
Poor past obstetric history.
Genetic factors.

Reassurance of patient, if there is no reduced foetal moments, normal FHR on auscultation and no risk factor. C

Further investigations should be carried out in women with reduced foetal movements or having risk factor for stillbirth.

7.2. What should be covered in clinical examination?

Examination
Height.
Weight.
Blood pressure.
Pallor.
Fundal height.
Amount of liquor.
Estimated foetal weight.
Foetal heart rate.

If the woman presents with reduced foetal movements, auscultate foetal heart rate using handheld Doppler device to exclude foetal death. B

Clinical assessment of woman with reduced foetal movement should include assessment of foetal size with the aim of detecting SGA foetus. B

If presence of foetal heartbeat is not confirmed, ultrasound, should be carried out.

7.3. What is the role of CTG?

CTG should be done in the woman over 28 weeks of gestation with confirmed reduced foetal movements to exclude foetal compromise at least for 20 minutes. B

Several studies have concluded that if the term foetus does not experience foetal heart rate acceleration for 80 minutes, a foetal compromise is likely to be present.

7.4. What is the role of ultrasound scanning?

Ultrasound features
Abdominal circumference.
Estimated foetal weight.
Amount of liquor.
Foetal morphology if not done before.

It is recommended to carry out ultrasound in the woman after 28 weeks of gestation if the woman presents with decreased foetal movements despite a normal CTG or if there are any additional risk factors for FGR/stillbirth preferably within 24 hours. B

This guideline recommended that both investigations, CTG and ultrasound, be performed within two hours if woman reported no foetal movements and within 12 hour if she reported reduced foetal movements. **(Evidence level 2-)**

A study concluded that women with reduced foetal movement but no additional pregnancy risk factors did not require further follow up once the CTG and the amniotic fluid volume is normal.

(Evidence level 2-)

7.5. Is there any role for the biophysical profile?

There may be a role for the selective use of BPP in the management or investigation of reduced foetal movement. B

Uncontrolled observational studies gave evidence that BPP has good negative predictive value; that foetal death is rare in the presence of normal BPP.

8. WHAT IS THE OPTIMAL SURVEILLANCE METHOD FOR WOMEN WHO HAVE PRESENTED WITH REDUCED FOETAL MOVEMENT IN WHOM INVESTIGATIONS ARE NORMAL?

Women should be reassured that 70% of pregnancies with a single episode of reduced foetal movement are uncomplicated. C

There is no data to support formal foetal movement counting after women have perceived reduced foetal movement with normal investigations. C

If a woman experiences further episodes of definite reduced foetal movement, she should immediately contact her doctor.

9. WHAT IS THE OPTIMAL MANAGEMENT OF WOMEN WHO PRESENTS RECURRENTLY WITH REDUCED FOETAL MOVEMENT?

When a woman recurrently perceives reduced foetal movement, her case should be reviewed to exclude predisposing causes. C

Women with recurrent episodes of reduce foetal movements should have her ultrasound done. B

A woman who presents on two or more occasions with reduced foetal movement is at increased risk of poor perinatal outcome compared with those who attend on only one occasion. ✓

10. WHAT IS THE OPTIMAL MANAGEMENT OF RFM BEFORE 24 WEEKS OF GESTATION?

Confirmation of foetal heart rate on Doppler hand held device.

If no movement is felt by 24 weeks then refer the patient to foetal specialist to rule out any foetal neuromuscular condition.

11. WHAT IS THE OPTIMAL MANAGEMENT OF RFM BETWEEN 24 AND 28 WEEKS?

Confirmation of foetal heart by hand held Doppler.

12. WHAT SHOULD WE DOCUMENT ON MATERNAL RECORDS?

It is important that full details of assessment and management are documented. It is also important to record the advice given about follow up and when and where to present if a further episode of reduced foetal movement is perceived.

79 Protocol Reduced Foetal Movements

Assessment

History: Gestational age, parity, duration of reduced foetal movements, number of foetal movements, any history of abdominal pain, vaginal leaking and bleeding, history of medical disorders, history of previous IUD and anomalous baby.

Identification of risk factors

Extreme maternal age.	Smoking.
Past poor obstetric history including IUD.	Recurrent episodes of reduced movements.
Hypertension.	IUGR.
Diabetes.	

Examination

Blood pressure, abdominal examination for fundal height, lie, presentation, liquor volume, estimated foetal weight and foetal heart rate, speculum examination if suspicion of leaking.

Investigations

CTG and obstetrical ultrasound (foetal heart rate, abdominal circumference, amount of liquor and estimated foetal weight) in every patient and in high risk patients, biophysical profile and Doppler are indicated.

Management

Keep patient for observation.

Foetal kick count chart (at least 10 movements in two hours).

Confirmation of foetal heart by ultrasonography.

< 24 weeks	**24–28 weeks**	**>28 weeks**
Confirmation of foetal heart rate. By Doppler hand held device. If no movement felt by 24 weeks, then refer to foetal specialist.	Confirmation of foetal heart rate. By Doppler hand held device. Also get an ultrasound done to confirm foetal heart rate and movements. Manage accordingly.	**In low risk:** (No risk factor for IUD or IUGR). Confirmation of foetal heart rate by Doppler hand held device—CTG. Ultrasound for AFI. If movements become normal and investigations are normal then reassure the patient and send her home. If the patient feels reduced foetal movements again, she should immediately report to hospital. **In high risk:** (Risk factor for IUD or foetal growth restriction). Confirmation of foetal heart rate by Doppler hand held device. Ultrasound CTG. Biophysical profile. Umbilical artery doppler. If reduced foetal movements settle and investigations are normal then observe patient for some time and send her home after reassurance and advise to report to hospital in case of repeat episode. If reduced foetal movements persist or investigations show some abnormality then manage accordingly in view of gestational age, risk factor and abnormality of investigations.

RECURRENT EPISODE OF REDUCE FOETAL MOVEMENTS

Admit patient. Foetal heart rate by sonic aid. Rule out any risk factor for IUD, IUGR. Foetal kick count. CTG. Ultrasound with biophysical profile and Doppler.	Counsel the patient regarding poor outcome of baby with repeated episode of reduce foetal movements. Steroid cover if required. Manage according to gestational age and investigations results.

Guideline 80
Shoulder Dystocia

Adapted from Green Top Guideline Number 42, March 2012

1. PURPOSE

The purpose of this guideline is to review the current evidence regarding the possible prediction, prevention and management of shoulder dystocia.

2. BACKGROUND

Shoulder dystocia is defined as requirement of additional obstetrical manoeuvres due to difficulty in delivery of the body of baby after the head has delivered and gentle traction has failed. Dystocia occurs when there is impaction of either foetal shoulder on the pubic symphysis or sacral promontory.

Incidence varies from 0.58%–0.70%. **(Evidence level 2+ and 3)**

There is significant perinatal morbidity and mortality associated with it. **(Evidence level 2+)**

Brachial plexus injury is one of the most common foetal complications of shoulder dystocia occurring in 2.3–16% cases. Most of brachial plexus injury resolves and only 10% results in permanent neurological damage. **(Evidence level 2+ and 3)**

Neural morbidity includes seizures, cerebral palsy and brachial plexus injury.
Clavicle and humeral fractures.
Perinatal mortality.

Shoulder dystocia is also associated with maternal morbidity. **(Evidence level 2+)**

Post partum haemorrhage.
Third and fourth degree perineal tear.
Uterine rupture.

3. PREDICTION

Risk factors should alert for the possibility of shoulder dystocia. D

Risk assessment predicts only 16% of shoulder dystocia. C

Infant of a diabetic woman has 2–3 fold increased risk of shoulder dystocia. **(Evidence level 2 + and 3)**

Pre labour risk factors for shoulder dystocia	**Intrapartum risk factors for shoulder dystocia**
Previous shoulder dystocia. Macrosomia >4.5 kg. Diabetes mellitus. Maternal body mass index >30 kg/m2. Induction of labour.	Prolonged first stage of labour. Secondary arrest. Oxytocin augmentation. Prolonged second stage of labour. Assisted vaginal delivery.

4. PREVENTION OF SHOULDER DYSTOCIA?

4.1. Management of suspected foetal macrosomia.

4.1.1. Does induction of labour prevent shoulder dystocia?

Induction of labour does not prevent shoulder dystocia in non-diabetic women with a suspected macrosomic foetus. D

Induction of labour at term can reduce the incidence of shoulder dystocia in women with gestational diabetes. B

4.1.2. Should elective caesarean section be recommended for suspected foetal macrosomia to prevent Brachial Plexus Injury (BPI)?

Elective caesarean section should be considered to reduce the potential morbidity for pregnancies complicated by pre-existing diabetes mellitus or gestational diabetes mellitus, regardless of treatment, with an estimated foetal weight of greater than 4.5 kg. D

4.2. What are the recommendations for future pregnancy? What is the appropriate mode of delivery for the woman with a previous episode of shoulder dystocia?

Either caesarean section or vaginal delivery can be appropriate after a previous shoulder dystocia. The decision should be made jointly by the patient and her doctor. D

The rate of shoulder dystocia is ten times higher in women with previous history of shoulder dystocia and recurrence is 1–25%. **(Evidence level 3)**

5. MANAGEMENT OF SHOULDER DYSTOCIA

5.1. What measures should be taken when shoulder dystocia is anticipated in labour?

All birth attendants should be aware of the methods for diagnosing shoulder dystocia and the techniques required to facilitate delivery.

5.2. How is shoulder dystocia diagnosed?

Birth attendant should routinely look for signs of shoulder dystocia.

Difficulty with delivery of the face and chin.

The head remaining tightly applied to the vulva or even retracting (turtle-neck sign).

Failure of restitution of the foetal head.

Failure of the shoulders to descend.

Routine traction in an axial direction can be used to diagnose shoulder dystocia but any other traction should be avoided. D

There is no prophylactic role of McRobert's manoeuvre before delivery of the foetal head. **(Evidence level 3)**

5.3. How should shoulder dystocia be managed?

First line

Shoulder dystocia should be managed systematically.

Call for help.

Fundal pressure should be avoided as it can cause neonatal complications and uterine rupture. D

McRoberts' manoeuvre (flexion and abduction of the maternal hips, positioning the maternal thighs on her abdomen) is a simple, rapid, associated with less complications and effective intervention (successful in 90% cases), should be performed first. D

Suprapubic pressure (from the side of foetal back in a downward and lateral direction) should be used to improve the effectiveness of the McRoberts' manoeuvre. D

An episiotomy is not always necessary and should only be carried out to create more space for internal vaginal manoeuvres. D

Avoid maternal pushing as it increases the impaction of shoulder.

5.3.1. What measures are undertaken if simple technique fails?

Second line:

Internal manoeuvres or all fours position should be used if the McRoberts manoeuvre fails. ✓

Internal rotation manoeuvres: Insert hand in sacral hollow of vagina and apply pressure on anterior or posterior aspect of the posterior shoulder. Pressure on the posterior aspect of shoulder has additional benefit of reducing diameter by adducting the diameter. If pressure on the posterior shoulder is unsuccessful then apply pressure on posterior aspect of anterior shoulder, adduct and rotate the shoulders into the oblique diameter. **(Evidence level 4)**

Delivering the posterior arm reduces the diameter of the foetal shoulders by the width of the arm. The foetal wrist should be grasped and the posterior arm should be gently withdrawn from the vagina in a straight line. **(Evidence level 3)**

There are no randomized comparative studies to compare these two manoeuvres.

Slim, mobile, without epidural woman and with single doctor is more likely for all four position rather than obese, non-mobile and with epidural that is more fit for internal manoeuvres so internal manoeuvres and all four position should be decided on individual basis. **(Evidence level 4)**

In the Pakistani setup, this method is not very popular.

5.3.2. What measures should be taken if first and second-line manoeuvres fail?

Third-line manoeuvres should be considered very carefully to avoid unnecessary maternal morbidity and mortality, particularly by inexperienced practitioners.

Third-line manoeuvres include:

Cleidotomy (surgical division of clavicle or bending by finger).

Symphysiotomy (dividing the anterior fibres of symphyseal ligament).

Zavanelli manoeuvre (vaginal placement of head and delivery by caesarean section).

5.4. What is the optimal management of the woman and baby after shoulder dystocia?

Birth attendants should be alert to the possibility of postpartum haemorrhage and severe perineal tears.

The baby should be examined by neonatologist for any injury.

6. RISK MANAGEMENT

6.1. Training

All maternity staff should participate in shoulder dystocia training at least annually. D

Practical shoulder dystocia training has been shown to improve knowledge, confidence and management of simulated shoulder dystocia. Training has also been shown to improve the actor patients' perception of their care during simulated shoulder dystocia.

6.2. What measures can be taken to ensure optimal management of shoulder dystocia?

Manoeuvre should be demonstrated in direct view, as they are complex and difficult to understand by description alone. Higher fidelity training equipment should be used.

6.3. Documentation

Documentation should be accurate and comprehensive.

It is important to record the following within the birth record:

Time of delivery of the head and time of delivery of the body.

Anterior shoulder at the time of the dystocia.

Manoeuvres performed, their timing and sequence.

Maternal perineal and vaginal examination.

Estimated blood loss.

Staff in attendance with names and the time they arrived.

Condition of the baby at delivery (Apgar score).

Umbilical cord blood acid-base measurements.

Neonatal assessment should be documented.

Document the position of the foetal head at delivery to facilitate identification of the anterior and posterior shoulder during the delivery.

Protocol 81
Shoulder Dystocia

Obstetrical emergency.	
Call for help.	
Two obstetrical teams—one for resuscitation and the other for management.	
PREREQUISITES	
Empty the bladder.	
Give adequate analgesia.	
Generous episiotomy (only as pre-emptive measure).	
PROCEDURE	
McRoberts manoeuvre This procedure involves flexing and abducting the maternal hips, positioning the maternal thighs up onto the maternal abdomen. This position flattens the sacral promontory and results in cephalad rotation of the pubic symphysis.	
Suprapubic pressure The hand of an assistant should be placed suprapubically over the foetal anterior shoulder, applying pressure in a cardiopulmonary resuscitation style with a downward and lateral motion on the posterior aspect of the foetal shoulder. This manoeuvre should be attempted while continuing downward traction.	
Internal rotation manoeuvres 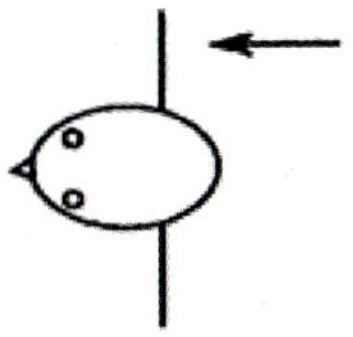 **Rubin II** At vaginal examination, apply pressure as indicated. If shoulders move into the oblique diameter, attempt delivery.	

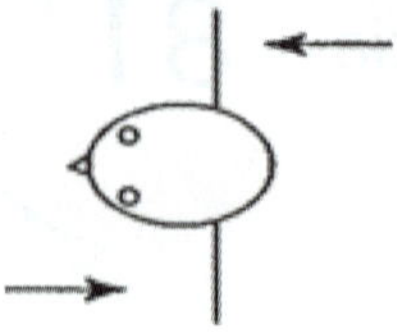 **Rubin II + Woods Corkscrew manoeuvre** If unsuccessful, add the Woods Corkscrew manoeuvre and continue rotation in the same direction. Use both hands and apply pressure as indicated. If shoulder now moves into the oblique, attempt delivery. If this is unsuccessful, continue rotation 180 degrees and deliver.	
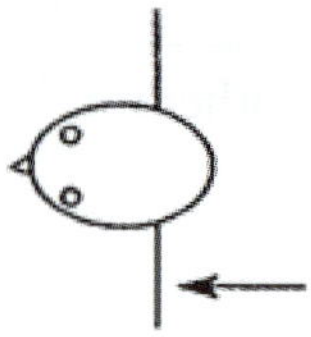 **Reverse Woods Corkscrew manoeuvre** If the last manoeuvre is unsuccessful, change to reverse Woods Corkscrew manoeuvre. Slide fingers down to back of posterior shoulder and attempt 180 degree rotation in the opposite direction Note: Rubin 1 = Suprapubic pressure.	
Removal of posterior arm Removal of the posterior arm involves placing the hand in the vagina and locating the foetal arm, which sometimes is displaced behind the foetus and must be nudged anteriorly. The foetal elbow is then flexed, and the forearm is delivered in a sweeping motion over the anterior chest wall of the foetus. The upper arm should never be grasped and pulled directly, because this step may result in a fracture of the humerus.	
Manoeuvres of last resort for shoulder dystocia a. **Deliberate clavicle fracture** Direct upward pressure on the mid-portion of the foetal clavicle; reduces the shoulder-to-shoulder distance. b. **Zavanelli manoeuvre** Cephalic replacement followed by caesarean delivery; involves rotating the foetal head into a direct occiput anterior position, then flexing and pushing the vertex back into the birth canal, while holding continuous upward pressure until caesarean delivery is accomplished.	

c. **General anaesthesia**

Musculoskeletal or uterine relaxation with halothane (Fluothane) or another general anaesthetic may bring about enough uterine relaxation to affect delivery. Oral or intravenous nitroglycerin may be used as an alternative to general anaesthesia.

d. **Abdominal surgery with hysterotomy**

General anaesthesia is induced and caesarean incision performed, after which the surgeon rotates the infant transabdominally through the hysterotomy incision, allowing the shoulders to rotate, much like a Woods Corkscrew manoeuvre. Another obstetrician then accomplishes vaginal extraction.

e. **Symphysiotomy**

Intentional division of the fibrous cartilage of the symphysis pubis under local anaesthesia. It should be used only when all other manoeuvres have failed and capability of caesarean delivery is unavailable.

DOCUMENTATION

Documentation of the management of shoulder dystocia should concentrate on the manoeuvres performed and the duration of the event. Other team members assisting the delivery should be listed, as well as cord pH, if obtained. Specific notation regarding which arm was impacted against the pubis should be made in the event that subsequent nerve palsy develops. The delivery should be reviewed with the parents, and the management and prognosis for any infant palsy should be explained.

DETAILS OF DOCUMENTATION

Timing is crucial

Onset of active labour.		Delivery of head.	
Start of second stage.		Time shoulder dystocia recognized.	
Delivery of infant.		Time help called.	
		Time between delivery of head and baby.	

ANTEPARTUM	
History: Prior shoulder dystocia, gestational diabetes, largest prior newborn birth weight.	
Estimated foetal weight in current pregnancy.	
Assessment of pelvis.	
INTRAPARTUM PROCEDURES	
Call for help to OBG team, paediatrics and anaesthesia team.	
Episiotomy extended.	
Hip flexion (McRoberts manoeuvre).	
Suprapubic pressure (stand on the side of the occiput).	
Delivery of posterior arm.	
Posterior scapula (Woods Cork Screw manoeuvre).	
All fours (Gaskin manoeuvre), anterior scapula (Rubin manoeuvre), Zavanelli manoeuvre, Caesarean section.	
INTRAPARTUM DOCUMENTATION	
Information on mode of delivery, assisted delivery, traction on vertex, fundal pressure applied or not.	
POSTPARTUM STEPS AND DOCUMENTATION	
Counselling of patient and family.	
Perineal assessment if third or fourth degree laceration.	
Monitored for postpartum haemorrhage.	
Lacerations and tears.	
Plan to monitor postpartum depression.	
NEONATAL CARE AND DOCUMENTATION	
Evidence of injury or asphyxia—Cord blood gases.	
Apgar scores.	
Birth weight.	
Close follow up of baby.	

Reference:

Shoulder dystocia. ACOG Practice Bulletin No. 40. American College of Obstetricians and Gynaecologists. Obstet Gynaecol 2002;100:1045–50.

Guideline
Prevention of Early-Onset Neonatal Group B Streptococcal Disease 82

Adapted from Green Top Guideline No. 30 June 2010

1. PURPOSE AND SCOPE

The purpose of this guideline is to provide guidance to obstetricians, midwives and neonatologists on the prevention of Early-Onset Neonatal Group B Streptococcal (EOGBS) disease.

2. BACKGROUND

Group B streptococcus (streptococcal agalactiae) is recognized as the most frequent cause of severe early-onset (at less than seven days of age) infection in newborn infants.

Less than 1% maternity units go for routine screening for Group B Streptococcal (GBS) infection during pregnancy in UK unlike other counties like USA and Canada. UK does not go for routine screening and Intrapartum Antibiotic Prophylaxis (IAP) as this is very costly, there are side effects of antibiotics and number of infants suffering from early onset GBS infection are same in UK and USA where they do routine screening and intrapartum antibiotic prophylaxis.

3. ANTENATAL SCREENING

3.1. Should all pregnant women be offered bacteriological screening for GBS?

Routine bacteriological screening of all pregnant women for antenatal GBS carriage is not recommendeduntil it is proven that screening does more good than harm and its benefits are more cost effective. D

3.2. If GBS is detected incidentally earlier in the pregnancy, should women be treated before the onset of labour?

Antenatal treatment with benzyl penicillin is not recommended but intrapartum antibiotic should be given in such cases. C

3.3. Should women be screened for GBS or receive intrapartum antibiotic prophylaxis if GBS was detected in a previous pregnancy?

Current evidence does not support screening for GBS infection or the administration of intrapartum antibiotic prophylaxis to women in whom GBS carriage was detected in a previous pregnancy. D

4. REDUCING THE RISK OF NEONATAL GBS DISEASE IN WOMEN KNOWN TO BE COLONIZED WITH GBS.

4.1. How should GBS bacteriuria in the current pregnancy be managed?

Clinician should offer intrapartum antibiotic prophylaxis to women with GBS bacteriuria identified during the current pregnancy. C

4.2. Should women receive intrapartum antibiotic prophylaxis if GBS is detected in the current pregnancy?

Intrapartum antibiotic prophylaxis should be offered if GBS is detected on a vaginal swab in the current pregnancy. C

4.3. How should women with known GBS colonization undergoing planned caesarean section be managed?

Antibiotic prophylaxis specific for GBS is not required for women undergoing planned caesarean section in the absence of labour and with intact membranesas the risk of neonatal early onset GBS disease is extremely low in this circumstance. C

4.4. How should women known to be colonized with GBS who experience spontaneous rupture of membranes at term be managed?

Immediate induction of labour and intrapartum antibiotic prophylaxis should be offered to all women with pre labour rupture of membranes at 37 weeks of gestation or more. D

4.5. How should women with GBS colonization and suspected chorioamnionitis be managed?

If chorioamnionitis is suspected, broad-spectrum antibiotic therapy including an agent active against GBS should replace GBS-specific intrapartum antibiotic prophylaxis and induction of labour should be considered. A

5. MANAGEMENT OF LABOUR (INCLUDING RUPTURE OF MEMBRANES) TO REDUCE THE RISK OF NEONATAL GBS DISEASE IN WOMEN WITHOUT KNOWN GBS COLONIZATION

5.1. Should women presenting in preterm labour with intact membranes be offered intrapartum antibiotic prophylaxis?

Women presenting with established preterm labour with intact membranes with no other risk factors for GBS should not routinely be offered intrapartum antibiotic prophylaxis unless they are known to be colonized, with GBS. C

5.2. How should women with clinical risk factors such as a pyrexia (>38°C) in labour be managed?

Intrapartum antibiotic prophylaxis should be offered to women who have pyrexia in labour, as it is a risk factor for early onset GBS disease. C

Women who have pyrexia in labour should be offered broad-spectrum antibiotics including an antibiotic for prevention of neonatal early onset GBS disease.

5.3. How should women with term prelabour rupture of membranes be managed?

The evidence of intrapartum antibiotic prophylaxis for women with the term prelabour rupture of membranes is unclear and NICE recommends that it is not given, unless there are other risk factors. C

Women with prelabour rupture of membranes at term should be offered immediate induction of labour or induction after 24 hours.

5.4. How should women with preterm prelabour rupture of membranes be managed to reduce the risk of neonatal GBS disease?

Antibiotic prophylaxis for GBS is unnecessary for women with preterm rupture of membranes without risk factor for GBS. C

5.5. Should women with a previous baby with neonatal GBS disease be offered IAP?

Intrapartum antibiotic prophylaxis should be offered to women with previous baby with neonatal GBS disease as there is increased chance of GBS in next baby. D

6. WHICH ANTIBIOTICS SHOULD BE GIVEN TO PREVENT EARLY-ONSET NEONATAL GBS DISEASE?

For women who have accepted intrapartum antibiotic prophylaxis, benzyl penicillin should be administered as soon as possible after the onset of labour and given regularly until delivery. B

It is recommended that 3 g intravenous benzyl penicillin be given as soon as possible after the onset of labour and 1.5 g 4-hourly until delivery. Clindamycin 900 mg should be given intravenously eitght hourly to those allergic to benzyl penicillin. Oral antibiotics for intrapartum antibiotic prophylaxis are not recommended because of variable absorption in labour. **(Evidence level 3)**

7. SHOULD VAGINAL CLEANSING BE PERFORMED IN LABOUR?

There is no evidence that intrapartum vaginal cleansing will reduce the risk of neonatal GBS disease. C

8. HOW SHOULD THE NEWBORN INFANT BE MANAGED?

8.1. How should well infants at risk of early onset GBS disease be monitored?

Well infants at risk of early onset GBS should be observed for the first 12–24 hours after birth with regular assessments of general wellbeing, feeding, heart rate, respiratory rate and temperature.

The great majority of infants (89–94%) who develop early onset GBS signs within the first 24 hours after birth have had one or more risk factor sevident in or before labour.

A significant number will also have had signs of foetal distress, an emergency delivery and low Apgar scores. Clearly, any baby with clinical signs and symptoms compatible with sepsis should be evaluated and commenced on antibiotics. Other infants without clinical signs but with other risk factors should be observed closely for such signs over the first 24 hours after birth.

8.2. Should postnatal antibiotic prophylaxis be given to low-risk term infants?

Postnatal antibiotic prophylaxis is not recommended for asymptomatic without known antenatal risk factors.	C
The argument for using prophylactic treatment in well infants is stronger in the presence of multiple maternal risk factors but is still unproven. However, in well infants whose mothers had risk factors and received appropriate intrapartum antibiotic prophylaxis, the risk of early onset GBS is significantly lower and these infants can be observed for 24 hours without treatment.	C
Infants with clinical signs of early onset GBS should be treated promptly with appropriate antibiotics.	C

8.3. How should the well infant with one or more risk factors be treated?

There is no sufficient evidence for clear treatment recommendations in well newborn infants with risk factors for GBS.	C

There are two schools of thought: some clinicians give antibiotics to a new born with risk factor for GBS but some observe the infant.	

8.4. How should the neonate with clinical signs of early onset GBS disease be managed?

Infants with clinical signs of early onset GBS should be treated promptly with appropriate antibiotics.

Blood cultures should always be obtained before antibiotic treatment is commenced, and cerebrospinal fluid cultures should be considered unless the clinical condition precludes a lumbar puncture. **(Evidence level 3)**

8.5. How should the infant of a mother with a previous infant with GBS disease be managed?

For a well infant whose mother has had a previous infant with GBS disease, either clinical evaluation after birth and observation for around 24 hours are necessary, or blood cultures need to be obtained and the infant treated with benzyl penicillin until the culture results are available. It is unclear whether further action is necessary for the well infant. C

8.6. Are routine neonatal surveillance cultures of value?

It is not necessary to perform routine surface cultures or blood cultures on well infants. ✓

Most infants who develop early onset GBS disease present with illness soon after birth and 90% have presented clinically by 24 hours of age, before culture results become available. **(Evidence level 3)**

8.7. Is there any need for breastfeeding to be avoided?

There is no evidence to discourage breastfeeding where there are concerns regarding the possible risk of transmission of GBS disease.

Protocol 83
Prevention of Early-Onset Neonatal Group B Streptococcal Disease

INDICATIONS FOR OFFERING GROUP B STREPTOCOCCAL SPECIFIC INTRAPARTUM ANTIBIOTIC PROPHYLAXIS	
Previous baby with GBS infection.	
GBS bacteriuria in the current pregnancy.	
Vaginal swab positive for GBS in current pregnancy.	
Pyrexia (>38 C) in labour (give broad spectrum antibiotics to include GBS cover).	
Chorioamnionitis.	
RISK FACTORS	
Intrapartum fever (>38 C).	
Prolonged rupture of membranes (>18 hours) at term.	
Prematurity (< 35 weeks of gestation).	
Positive GBS swab in previous pregnancy.	
Positive GBS swab in current pregnancy.	
ANTENATAL SCREENING FOR GBS	
Routine bacteriological screening of all pregnant women in antenatal is not recommended. Antenatal treatment with benzyl penicillin is not recommended.	
Antibiotic prophylaxis specific for GBS is not required for women undergoing planned C-Section.	
Immediate induction of labour and intrapartum antibiotic prophylaxis is offered to all women with prelabour rupture of membranes at 37 week gestation or more.	
INTRAPARTUM MANAGEMENT	
Women presenting with preterm labour with intact membranes with no risk factor for GBS should not be routinely offered intrapartum antibiotic prophylaxis.	

Intrapartum antibiotic prophylaxis should be offered to women who have pyrexia in labour (temp >38 C), history of previous baby with GBS, GBS bacteriuria in current pregnancy or colonized with GBS.	
Women with prelabour rupture of membranes at term should be offered immediate induction of labour or induction after 24 hours.	
Intrapartum antibiotic prophylaxis should be administered as soon as possible after the onset of labour and given regularly until delivery (3 g I/V benzyl penicillin after onset of labour and 1.5 g x four hourly until delivery). Oral antibiotics are not recommended.	
POSTNATAL MANAGEMENT	
Infants at risk of early onset GBS should be observed for the first 12 to 24 hours after birth with regular assessment of general well being, feeding, heart rate, R/R and temperature.	
Infants with clinical signs of early onset GBS should be treated promptly with appropriate antibiotics.	
There is no need to discourage breastfeeding regarding possible risk of transmission of GBS disease.	

Guideline 84
Tocolysis in Preterm Labour

Adapted from Green Top Guideline No.1b, February 2011

1. BACKGROUND

Preterm birth is defined as birth at less than 37+6 weeks of gestation.

Preterm births can be classified into:

Mild preterm birth: 32weeks–36+6 weeks.

Very preterm: 28weeks–31+6 weeks.

Extremely preterm: 24weeks–27+6 weeks.

Risk of death or neurosensory disability increases with decreasing gestational age.

Prevention and treatment of preterm birth is important. Currently various agents are used in suppressing uterine contractions which include beta-agonists, calcium channel blockers, oxytocin receptor antagonists, prostaglandin synthetase inhibitors, nitric oxide donors and magnesium sulphate.

2. PURPOSE

This guideline provides information regarding effectiveness and safety of tocolytic drugs for treatment of preterm labour.

3. USES OF TOCOLYSIS FOR WOMEN IN PRETERM LABOUR

3.1. Does tocolysis prevent preterm birth?

Use of a tocolytic drug is associated with a prolongation of pregnancy for up to seven days but with no significant effect on preterm birth and no clear effect on perinatal or neonatal morbidity.

There is no clear evidence that tocolytic drugs improve outcome but provide time for completing a course of corticosteroids or in utero transfer. A

3.2. Does the use of any tocolytic drug prevent perinatal or neonatal death and neonatal morbidity?

Use of a tocolytic drug is not associated with a clear reduction in perinatal or neonatal mortality, or neonatal morbidity. A

4. WHEN SHOULD TOCOLYTIC DRUG BE USED?

Tocolysis may be considered for women with suspected preterm labour who have had an otherwise uncomplicated pregnancy. B

Any contraindication to prolonging pregnancy is a contraindication to tocolytic therapy. ✓

ABSOLUTE CONTRAINDICATIONS	RELATIVE CONTRAINDICATION
Congenital and chromosomal abnormalities.	Minor placenta previa.
Severe preeclampsia.	Non reactive CTG.
Placental abruption.	Foetal growth restriction.
Intrauterine infection.	Multiple gestation.
Foetal compromise.	
Advance cervical dilatation.	
Placental insufficiency.	

As currently there is no evidence that tocolysis has benefit for baby so decision regarding tocolysis should be taken in liaison with parents and senior obstetrician should take decision regarding tocolysis.

5. IS ONE TOCOLYTIC DRUG MORE EFFECTIVE IN PREVENTING PRETERM BIRTH THAN ANOTHER?

Nifedipine and atosiban (not available in Pakistan) have comparable effectiveness in delaying birth for up to seven days. A

Compared with beta-agonists, nifedipine is associated with improvement in neonatal outcome, although there are no long-term data. A

Ritodrine and atosiban are licensed for the treatment of threatened preterm labour. Although nifedipine is not licensed for use in preterm labour but it is widely used due to its low cost, availability in Pakistan and oral administration. Ritodrine is not widely use these days due to its side effects.

6. WHAT ARE THE COMPARATIVE ADVERSE EFFECTS FOR THE WOMEN OF ALTERNATIVE TOCOLYTIC DRUGS FOR PRETERM LABOUR?

Beta agonists have high frequency of side effects as compared to nifedipine, atosiban and COX inhibitors but how they compare with each other is unclear. A

Nifedipine is contraindicated in cardiac disease and should be used with caution with diabetes or multiple pregnancies.

Adverse effects of Atosiban.	**Adverse effects of β agonists.**	**Adverse effects of calcium channel blockers.**
Nausea.	Palpitations.	Blockers.
Vomiting.	Tremors.	Flushing .
Chest pain.	Nausea or vomiting.	Palpitations.
Dyspnoea.	Headache.	Nausea.
Injection site reactions.	Chest pain.	Vomiting.
	Dyspnoea.	Hypotension.
	Pulmonary oedema.	
	Palpitations.	
	Tremors.	

Using more than one type of tocolytic in combination with another appears to increase the risk of adverse effects and so should be avoided. B

7. WHAT ARE THE COMPARATIVE EFFECTS FOR THE BABY OF ALTERNATIVE TOCOLYTIC DRUGS FOR PRETERM LABOUR?

They are unclear. B

Calcium channel blockers associate with less neonatal respiratory distress syndrome, necrotising enterocolitis and intraventricular haemorrhage. **(Evidence level 1+)**

Nifedipine, the most commonly used calcium channel blocker, crosses the placenta but its long term effects on child is unclear. **(Evidence level 2+)**

The oxytocin receptor agonist atosiban is associated with an increase in birth weight. **(Evidence level 1–)**

COX inhibitors cross the placenta and result into premature closure of ductus arteriosus with consequent pulmonary hypertension, persistent patent ductus arteriosus, necrotising enterocolitis and intraventricular haemorrhage.

Magnesium sulphate was associated with an increased risk of foetal, neonatal and infant death. **(Evidence level 1+)**

8. WHAT ARE THE RECOMMENDED DOSAGE REGIMENS FOR NIFEDIPINE AND ATOSIBAN?

Nifedipine—Initial oral dose of 20 mg followed by 10–20 mg, three to four times daily, adjusted according to uterine activity for up to 48 hours with a total dose of 60 mg. ✓

A suggested dose of atosiban is an initial bolus dose of 6.75 mg over one minute, followed by an infusion of 18 mg/hour for three hours, then 6 mg/hour for up to 45 hours (to a maximum of 330 mg). ✓

There is no clear consensus on the ideal dosage regimen for nifedipine when used for tocolysis.

9. WHAT IS THE COST EFFECTIVENESS OF TOCOLYSIS FOR PRETERM LABOUR?

The purchase price of atosiban is ten times higher than nifedipine.

10. SHOULD TOCOLYSIS BE USED IN MULTIPLE PREGNANCIES?

There is no specific evidence for a beneficial role of tocolytic drugs in preterm labour in multiple pregnancies. ✓

11. IS MAINTAINANCE TOCOLYTIC THERAPY WORTHWHILE?

Maintenance therapy is not recommended. B

85 Protocol Tocolysis in Preterm Labour

PROTOCOL FOR TOCOLYSIS IN PRETERM LABOUR	
Diagnosis of preterm labour	
Regular uterine contractions with progressive changes in cervix.	
Cervical dilatation > 1 cm.	
Cervical effacement >50%.	
INVESTIGATIONS	
All baseline investigations.	
For bacterial vaginosis.	
Screening for foetal fibronectin.	
TREATMENT	
Tocolysis.	
Corticosteroids for foetal lung maturity.	
Treatment of infection if any.	
AIM OF TOCOLYSIS	
Allow in utero transfer to facility with neonatal intensive care unit.	
Allow time for administration of corticosteroids.	
TOCOLYTIC AGENTS	
Calcium channel blockers (Nifedipine).	

Oxytocin receptor antagonists (Atosiban).	
Betamimetics (terbutaline, ritodrine).	
Magnesium sulphate.	
Nitric oxide donor (nitroglycerine patch).	
Prostaglandin synthetase inhibitors.	
DOSAGE AND ROUTES OF ADMINISTRATION	
Calcium channel blocker (nifedipine): Initial oral dose of 20 mg followed by 10–20 mg, three to four times daily, adjusted according to uterine activity for up to 48 hours.	
Oxytocin receptor antagonists (Atosiban): Not available in Pakistan.	
Betamimetics (terbutaline, ritodrine): Terbutaline 0.25 mg, subcutaneously every 20 minutes to three hours.	
Ritodrine: Initial dose 50–100 microgram/min. I/V increased @50 microgram/min every 10 minutes. until contractions cease or side effects develop.	
Magnesium sulphate: Loading dose 4 gm as a slow bolus over 15–30 minutes. Maintenance dose 1 gm/hour for 24 hours. Stop if side effects occur (resp. rate<12, B.P drops, loss of patellar reflex, urine o/p <100 ml in four hours).	
Nitric oxide donor (nitroglycerine patch): 10 mg patch for every 12 hour, continue until contraction ceases upto 48 hours.	
Prostaglandin synthetase inhibitors (indomethacin): Loading dose, 50 mg rectally or 50–100 mg orally then 25–50 mg orally every six hours for 48 hours.	
DRUG OF CHOICE	
Calcium channel blocker (nifedipine) is the drug of choice because it is cost effective, easily available and with less side effects.	

FOETO-MATERNAL MONITORING WHEN NIFEDIPINE IS USED	
Maternal pulse, BP, uterine contractions should be monitored every 30 minutes.	
Foetal heart rates should be monitored every 30 minutes.	
DOCUMENTATION	
Drug used should be clearly mentioned alongwith dosage and route of administration in patient's medical record.	

Bibliography

1. Baker PN, Kenny L. 2011. *Obstetrics by Ten Teachers*. 19th edition. New York. CRC Press.
2. Gilstrap III LC, Cunningham FG, Vandorsten JP. 2002. *Operative obstetrics*. second edition. McGraw Hill Companies.
3. Rock JA, Jones III HW. 2011. *TeLinde's Operative Gynaecology*. 10th edition. Lippincott Williams and Wilkins.
4. *RCOG Green Top guidelines*. Available: www.rcog.org.uk.
5. Wilcox SR. 2013. *Hyperemesis Gravidarum in Emergency Medicine Medication*. Medscape. Available at: emedicine.medscape.com/article/796564-medication
6. Ogonyemi DA. 2014. *Hyperemesis Gravidarum Treatment and Management*. Medscape. Available at: emedicine.medscape.com/article/254751–treatment.
7. *Induction of Labour. Guidance and all Guidelines, NICE*. July 2008. Available at; www.nice.org.uk/guidance/cg70.
8. *The Management of Severe Pre-Eclampsia/Eclampsia: Care of the patient*. March 2006. RCOG Guideline no. 10 A. Available at: www.neonatalformulary.com/...guidelines/MAGNESIUM-SULPHATE-R.
9. *Labetalol—Care of the Obstetrical Patient Receiving I/V Labetalol for Hypertensive Disorders of Pregnancy. The Confidential Enquiry into Maternal and Child Health (CEMACH) 2007*.Available at: www.learningace.com/.../labetalol-care-of-the-obstretrical-patient-receivi.
10. *Care of the Obstetrical Patient Receiving Labetalol; Hypertensive Disorders of Pregnancy*. Australian Product Prescription Guide (APPG)
11. *Care of the Obstetrical Patient Receiving Labetalol; Hypertensive Disorders of Pregnancy*. The management of severe pre-eclampsia/eclampsia. RCOG Guideline No. 10A March 2006.
12. *Hypertension in Pregnancy: The Management of Hypertensive Disorders during Pregnancy*. NICE Guidelines. August 2010. Available at : http://www.nice.org.uk/guidance/cg107

13. *Gowning and gloving technique*—University of Illinois. Available at; chicago.medicine.uic.edu/.../UIC%20Gowning %20 and %20 Gloving.PDF‹

14. WHO Reproductive Health Library. *Misoprostol for cervical ripening and induction of labour*. Available at apps.who.int/rhl/pregnancy_childbirth/induction/CD000941.../en/‹

15. *Misoprostol Recommended Dosages* 2012-FIGO. Available at; wwww.figo.org/.../Misoprostol_Recommended%20Dosages%202012.pd

16. Cervical ripening ... IJGO, 2007 d *WHO recommendations for induction of labour*, 2011 e FIGO Guidelines: Prevention of PPH with misoprostol, 2012.

17. *Nifedipine Administration for Tocolysis; Tocolysis for women in preterm labour*. National guideline. Available at; www.guideline.gov

18. *Induction of labour*. ACOG Practice Bulletin No. 107.American College of Obstetricians and Gynaecologists. Obstet Gynaecol2009; 114:386–97.

19. *Vaginal birth after previous caesarean delivery*. Committee Opinion No. 115.American College of Obstetricians and Gynaecologists. Obstet Gynaecol 2010;116:450–63. Available at: www.acog.org/goto/PBListOfTitles.asp

20. *Patient safety in the surgical environment*. Committee Opinion No. 464.American College of Obstetricians and Gynaecologists. Obstet Gynaecol 2010;116:786–90. Available at: www.acog.org/-/.../Committee%20Opinions/Committee%20on%20Patient%

21. Committee on Obstetric Practice. *Antimicrobial prophylaxis for Caesarean delivery: timing of administration*. Committee Opinion No. 465.American College of Obstetricians and Gynaecologists. Obstet Gynaecol 2010;116:791–2.

22. *Fetal lung maturity*. ACOG Practice Bulletin No. 97.American College of Obstetricians and Gynaecologists. Obstet Gynaecol 2008;112:717–26.

23. Hobel CJ, Hyvarinen MA et al. *Prenatal and intrapartum high-risk screening*. Am J Obstet Gynaecol. 1973; 117: 1–9. PMID: 4722373

24. Shaw RW, Soutter WP, Stanton SL. 2008. *Shaw's Textbook of Gynaecology*. 14th edition. London. Elsevier.

25. Robert K. Stoelting,

26. Royal College of Obstetricians and Gynaecologists . *Management of HIV in pregnancy, Green Top Guideline* No. 30 June 2010. Available at:www.rcog.org.uk/...guidance/management-hiv-pregnancy-green-top-39

27. Royal College of Obstetricians and Gynaecologists. *Maternal collapse in pregnancy and the puerperium; Green-top Guideline* No.56. Available at: https://www.rcog.org.uk/globalassets/documents/guidelines/gtg56.pdf
28. Royal College of Obstetricians and Gynaecologists. *Obstetric cholestasis; Green Top Guideline* No 43, April 2011. Available at: www.rcog.org.uk/womens...guidance/obstetric-cholestasis-green-top-43
29. Royal College of Obstetricians and Gynaecologists. *Operative vaginal delivery; Green-top Guideline* No.26, July 2011. Available at: www.rcog.org.uk/...guidance/operative-vaginal-delivery-green-top-26
30. Keith Edmonds. February 2012. *Dewhurst's Textbook of Obstetrics and Gynaecology*, 8th Edition. Wiley-Blackwell
31. ACOG Committee on Practice Bulletins: Obstetrics. ACOG Practice Bulletin No. 80: *Premature rupture of membranes. Clinical management guidelines for obstetrician-gynaecologists.* Obstetrics and Gynaecol. 2007 Apr: 109(4): 1007–19.
32. Royal College of Obstetricians and Gynaecologists. *Preterm Prelabour Rupture of Membranes (PPROM); Green-top Guideline* no 44, October 2010. Available at : www.ranzcog.edu.au/doc/rcog-preterm-rupture-of-membranes.html
33. Royal College of Obstetricians and Gynaecologists. 2011. *Reduced Fetal Movements; Adapted from Green Top Guideline* Number 57. Available at: www.rcog.org.uk/...guidance/reduced-fetal-movements-green-top-57.
34. Royal College of Obstetricians and Gynaecologists. March 2012. *Shoulder dystocia; Adapted from Green Top Guideline* Number 42. Available at: www.rcog.org.uk/womens...guidance/shoulder-dystocia-green-top-42.
35. Politi S, Emidio LD, Cignini P et al. *Shoulder dystocia: an evidence based approach*. Journal of Prenatal Medicine. 2010 Jul-Sept; 4(3): 35–42.
36. F. Cunningham Kenneth Leveno Steven Bloom Catherine Y. Spong Jodi Dashe. 2014 *Williams' Obstetrics*. 24th Edition. Mc Graw Hill.
37. *Shoulder dystocia: an evidence based approach*. Journal of Prenatal Medicine ACOG Practice Bulletin No. 40. American College of Obstetricians and Gynaecologists. Obstet Gynaecol 2002; 100: 1045–50.

38. Money D, Allen VM. October 2013. *The prevention of early onset neonatal group B streptococcal disease*. SOGC Clinical Practice Guideline No. 298.
39. Royal College of Obstetricians and Gynaecologists. February 2011. *Tocolysis for woman in preterm labour; Green Top Guideline* No.1b. NHS Evidence. Available at://www.rcog.org.uk/globalassets/.../guidelines/gtg1b26072011.pdf
40. *Patient's Safety Checklist*. ACOG-American College of Obstetricians and Gynaecologists. Available at: www.acog.org › Resources and Publications
41. Cunningham F, Leveno K, Bloom S et al. 2014. *William's Obstetrics*. 24th edition. McGraw Hill Companies.
42. Edmonds DK. 2007. *Dewhurst's Textbook of Obstetrics and Gynaecology*. 7th edition. London. Blackwell Publishing.
43. Hatcher RA, Rinehart W, Blackburn R et al. 1997. *The Essentials of Contraceptive Technology*. Baltimore. John Hopkins University School of Public Health, Population Information Programme.
44. Department of Reproductive Health, World Health Organization. 2010. *Medical eligibility criteria for contraceptive use*. Fourth edition
45. James DK et al. 2010. *High Risk Pregnancy: Management Options*. 4th edition. St. Louis. Elseviers Saunders.
46. Khan YL, Khan RL. 2011. *Rashid Latif Text book of Gynaecology*. 6th edition. Paramount Publishers
47. Das K. 2005. *Clinical Methods in Surgery*. 3rd edition.
48. Walker BR et al. 2014. *Davidson's principles and practice of medicine*. 22nd edition. Churchill Livingstone Elsevier.
49. Douglas G, Nicol EF, Robertson CE. 2013. *Macleod's Clinical Examination*. 13th edition. Churchill Livingstone.
50. Butterworth JF, Mackey DC, Wasnick JD. 2013. *Clinical anaesthesiology*. 5th edition. USA. McGraw Hill Companies.
51. UNICEF. April 2013. *Breastfeeding on the worldwide agenda*. Available at: www.unicef.org/eapro/breastfeeding_on_worldwide_agenda.pdf
52. *Infection prevention guidelines for health care facilities–USAID*. Available at; pdf.usaid.gov/pdf_docs/PNACT433.pdf